CHINESE PATENT MEDICINES

A BEGINNER'S GUIDE

Mark Taylor
California Licensed Acupuncturist
National Board Certified Chinese Herbalist (NCCAOM)

Chinese Patent Medicines: A Beginner's Guide
Global Eyes International Press
343 Soquel Ave., #92
Santa Cruz, CA 95062
Copyright © 1998 by Mark Taylor.
All rights reserved. Printed in the United States of America
by Community Printers, Santa Cruz, CA.

Cover and interior design/production by Marianne Wyllie
Edited by Jeff Troiano
All photographs © by Mark Taylor, except those showing
Plum Flower packaging, courtesy of Mayway Corporation.

This book is intended to provide general information only.
The author is not giving medical advice or prescribing
medical treatments. The purpose of this book is to help
readers understand the nature of herbal treatments and to
assist them with health care questions. For any medical situation, please see your licensed health care practitioner.
The author and publisher assume no responsibility for an
individual's actions.

ISBN 0-9662973-0-X

This book is dedicated to my teachers,
who opened the door of herbal knowledge for me.

Dr. Sharon Feng
Dr. Jeffrey Pang
Dr. Janna Chow
Dr. Richard Liao
Dr. Lucy Hu

TABLE OF CONTENTS

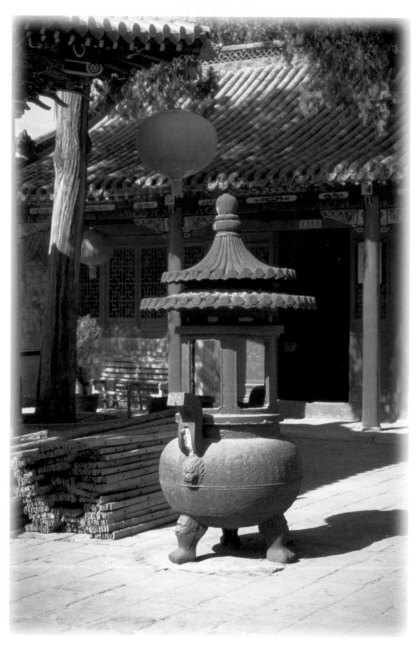

Temple of the Medicine God, Anguo

PREFACE

My purpose in writing this book is simple. I would like to make information regarding good quality Chinese Patent Medicines accessible to those who have no formal training in Chinese Medicine.

What are Chinese Patent Medicines? Simply put, "Patent Medicines" are herbal prescriptions, most often classic herb formulas from Traditional Chinese Medicine (TCM), produced in pill form so that they are available to the general public.

Most books written on the subject of Chinese Medicine are difficult to understand because of the terminology. Before I became a student of Chinese Medicine, I tried to read many of these texts and did not find them very useful.

This beginner's guide to Chinese Patent Medicines is simply a tool. A number of the formulas found in this book are extremely complex, and can only be understood clearly by a doctor of Chinese Medicine. I have chosen to describe only those elements of these formulas which could be useful to someone with little training in Chinese Medicine. The idea is to provide a common understanding, so that people can use herbal medicine to treat themselves without having to see a doctor.

Additionally, I would like to encourage an improvement in the quality of herbal products imported into the United States. Some excellent, quality-conscious Chinese factories produce some of the finest herbal medicine in the world. On the other hand, there are factories that produce counterfeit products that copy the images and reputations of the best factories. Other products, containing illegal drugs and other contaminants, are smuggled into this country every day and are sold to unsuspecting consumers.

In this book, I'll identify the best products of Chinese Herbal Medicine and provide the most current information on popular products sold both here and in China. As a retailer of natural foods and quality herbal products for the past 20 years, I have become quite familiar with most of the products sold in the marketplace. Over the years, I've worked diligently to increase my knowledge of the production values of herbal products manufactured in China and in other countries.

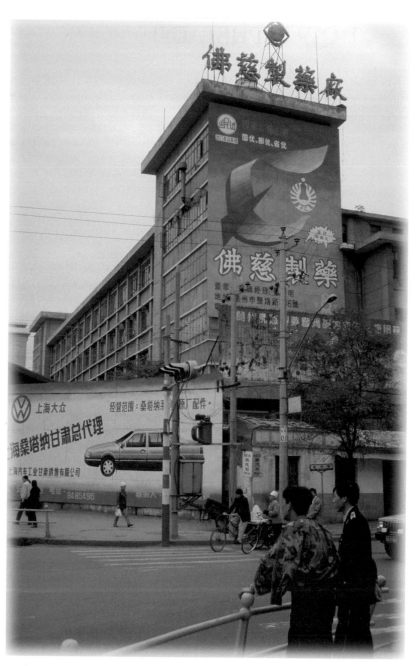

Lanzhou Foci Factory

HOW TO USE THIS BOOK

This book is intended to be used as a reference: 1. To explain the medicinal uses of Chinese Patent Medicines and 2. To provide accurate information so the reader can select the highest quality products on the market.

The first section of this book gives a brief background on the history of herbal medicine, in part to inform the reader about the benefits of Chinese Herbal Medicines, but also to put in perspective the politics involved in "alternatives" to Western-style Medicine and some of the problems with Chinese Patent Medicines.

Even more important, one of the main goals of this book is to explain to the reader the importance of good manufacturing procedures in the production of herbal medicine.

The main body of the text provides a detailed explanation of more than one hundred formulas which are very popular and widely used both here in the U.S., Asia, and in China. The following explains how to read the formula descriptions:

1. Yu Ping Feng San Wan   Classic Chinese name for the herb formula
2. Jade Screen Powder Pills   Translation of its meaning
3. The Teachings of Zhu Dan-Xi   Historical source of the formula
4. (Dan Xi Xin Fa)   Source book in Pinyin
5. Dr. Zhu Dan-Xi, 1481 A.D.   Name of the author and the date of the book

6. In some cases, I may include a caution about certain formulas. It may be a warning that some products are available in counterfeit form or a warning, for example, that the product might adversely affect a pregnancy.

Warning: This formula should not be taken by anyone who has heat signs, such as hot flashes, low grade fever, hot palms and soles of the feet or flushed face. (This warning is for Shi Chuan Da Bu Wan, see page 101.)

Caution: This product is widely counterfeited. (This is a commonly listed warning on a number of products.)

7. On the following line, I list the common uses of the formula. This often only provides a starting point for understanding, since the uses of some prescriptions need explanation.

Common Usage: Frequent common colds, allergies.

8. In this section, I present a simplified explanation, often in Western terms, so that a reader who doesn't understand Chinese Medicine will grasp the idea behind the formula.

Description: This three-herb formula boosts a deficient, weak immune system which makes an individual vulnerable to a common cold, flu, and allergies. It can be used to promote the immune system, or to combat immune suppressed conditions such as Chronic Fatigue Syndrome or Epstein-Barr.

9. Here, I try to explain the thinking of Chinese doctors as they might diagnose a complaint from a patients. This is often a basic TCM textbook explanation of the complaint as it might be learned in a school of Traditional Chinese Medicine.

Chinese Diagnosis: An individual who is frequently sick or suffers from allergies has a Wei Qi (defensive or protective Qi) deficiency. Wei Qi protects the body from external evils (pathogens such as bacteria, viruses, and allergens). Wei Qi is the body's first line of defense against any infectious disease. A person with deficient Wei Qi more easily catches cold, more frequently catches colds, and is more susceptible to allergies, such as hay fever.

10. Finally, the book provides an explanation of the function of the individual herbs in the formula. In some instances, I may go into more detail regarding the role of an individual herb in a particular formula or I may explain some unique aspect of the treatment.

Ingredients in the Formula:

Huang Qi (astragalus root) promotes the body's overall energy, strengthening both digestion and the body's surface Qi (Wei Qi), which is controlled by the lungs. The body derives nutrients from food and then transforms that food into Qi which is carried to the lungs where it is dispersed throughout the body. In order to protect the body, the lungs send out Wei Qi to the skin layer where it provides defense from external evils. It also protects the exterior of the body from wind and cold.

Bai Zhu (atractylodes rhizome) strengthens digestion. When digestion is strong, the body extracts nutrients effectively and will be better able to resist disease. This herb focuses on the need to replenish the protective energy of the body so that it does not become easily depleted. Bai Zhu also stabilizes the exterior of the body and protects the body from wind and cold.

Fang Feng (siler; ledebouriella root) guards against wind which carries pathogens and allergens such as dust, pollen and animal dander. The name Fang Feng literally translates to mean "guard against wind," thus protecting the body from wind-borne disease.

Unlike Western medicine which sees allergies as an aversion to particular substances, such as an allergic reaction to dairy products or a sneezing reaction to a particular type of pollen, Chinese Medicine looks to strengthen resistance and to improve digestion as a means of combating external evils. When the body is sufficiently strong, it will not be affected by colds or pollen allergens.

11. At the end of the individual herb explanation, I may offer a special note, information that I feel is valuable for the reader to know.

Note: It may take time, perhaps as long as a month, before some effects can be seen from taking Jade Screen Powder, such as less frequent and less severe colds and perhaps as long as five months before full effects are seen. Herbal products are not like drugs which rely on immediate results. Herbs work slowly and heal over time to provide lasting results, often without nasty side effects. Unlike antihistamine drugs, herb formulas that reduce allergic reactions do not cause drowsiness and impaired motor functioning.

12. Finally, I give the recommended dosage of an individual product.

Dosage: 8 pills three times per day.

ABOUT CHINESE TRANSLATION

There are different systems to translate the Chinese language. The two most commonly used systems of transliteration (the rendering of Chinese characters into English letters) are the old British system, Wade-Giles, and pinyin, which is the official system of the current Chinese government.

What does this mean to you? For a long time, for example, Peking was the official translation of the name of the Chinese capital, but Peking is the transliteration using the British system which, being politically associated with imperialism, is no longer officially used in China. Beijing is now the preferred translation because it is transliterated using the official pinyin system. Other examples of the differences between the systems of translation are Lanchow/Lanzhou; Tientsin/Tianjin; Kwangchow/Guangzhou.

Below are examples of the same formulas, using two different translations:

Shi Chuan Da Bu Wan
Shi Quan Da Bu Wan
Shih Chuan Ta Pu Wan

Zhi Bai Di Huang Wan
Chih Pai Di Huang Wan

Long Dan Xie Gan Wan
Lung Tan Xie Gan Wan

ABOUT HERB NAMES

Some names of formulas contain words like tang, pian, wan, and san. Often, these are part of the original herb formula name, such as Yin Qiao San (Honeysuckle and Forsythia Powder). Below, you will find translations of some of the common designations associated with Chinese Patent Medicines.

Tang

literally means herbal soup. Most herb prescriptions were formulated using bulk herbs which were cooked together like a soup. Traditionally, patients saw a Chinese Doctor who made a prescription by mixing together loose herbs. The patient took the herbs home and brewed it up as a tea.

San

means powder. Some prescriptions called for powdering loose herbs and then adding hot water, or in some cases adding honey to the powder to make herbal pills.

Wan

are small pills, usually black, now made by reducing the water content of the tang (herbal soup) until the pill is firm and solid. An example is Si Wu Tang Wan, page 179.

Herbal Pills made in China before the Twentieth Century were produced by combining herbs with water, honey, rice paste, wax, or flour. These pills were formed into solid spheres for easier long-term storage and handling.

Pian

is a larger pill, more the size of vitamin pills sold in Health Food stores in the U.S. Pian are manufactured by freeze-drying the herbal soup mixture (tang) and then tableting it, using standard manufacturing techniques with fillers, binders, and excipients (the materials added to the freeze-dried herbs to make the tableting efficient). An example is Lien Qiao Pai Du Pian, page 217.

Su

are concentrated pills. The active ingredient is concentrated by modern methods to increase the potency. An example is Huang Lian Su, pages 165, 235.

Chong Ji

are water soluble granules. It comes in packets which are intended to be consumed after adding hot water. It is taken like tea and is better suited for children who won't swallow pills. See Gan Mao Tui Re Chong Ji, page 233.

INTRODUCTION

The idea for this book occurred to me while I was doing research on Chinese Medicine. In the course of my research, I was surprised by the long, historical record of Chinese Herbal Medicine. The earliest known book that still survives, *Prescriptions for 52 Diseases (Wu Shi Er Bing Fang),* dates back to a period as early as the eighth century B.C. Even though some scholars estimate that Chinese Medicine has probably existed for more than 10,000 years, the historical record provides concrete documentation of nearly 3,000 years of continuous use.

Advocates of Western Medicine often denigrate Chinese Herbal Medicine and argue that it is not "scientific." They imply that it is folk medicine from the dark ages which should be discarded because it is not "modern" and "new." The illusion that has been fostered in the 20th century Western world is that anything "scientific" or "newly discovered" must be superior to everything that came before it, that the only knowledge of value is knowledge derived during the past 50 years.

In reality, medicine that has little effect and doesn't improve a patient's symptoms will disappear from the marketplace in a very short time simply because it doesn't work. If a treatment is ineffective, it will not be continued. It is my argument that any Chinese herbal treatment that has existed for several hundred years is effective and has proven its effectiveness in the experience of thousands—if not millions—of patients and doctors. I feel that this is a far tougher standard than the testing of a few hundred rats in a laboratory.

Before I became a student of Chinese Medicine, I had been using Chinese Herbal Medicine for several years. I was convinced of its value by my own experience with herb remedies. This inspired me to enroll as a student and to become a doctor of Chinese Medicine myself. Since returning to school, I have received a Master's Degree in Traditional Chinese Medicine and am currently a licensed acupuncturist today, practicing Chinese Medicine in Santa Cruz, California.

THE HISTORY OF CHINESE HERBAL MEDICINE

No one knows exactly when the first herbal materia medica appeared. *The Divine Peasant's Herbal (Shen Nong Ben Cao Jing),* reputed at one time to be the first known book to document individual herbs, probably appeared before 200 B.C. At about the same time, *The Yellow Emperor's Classic of Medicine (Huang Di Nei Jing)* appeared. The *Nei Jing,* as it is commonly called, is the text on which much of modern Traditional Chinese Medicine is based. About 400 years later, in 219 A.D., Dr. Chang's *Discussion of Cold Induced Disorders (Shang Han Lun)* appeared; it is the first surviving text that demonstrates the sophistication of Chinese Herbal Medicine. And it a testament to that book that, almost seventeen centuries later, the prescriptions first appearing in Dr. Chang's book are still in use today in clinics and hospitals throughout China. They remain the cornerstone on which herbal medicine is based. A large number of these same prescriptions are described in this book.

Many books on herbal medicine followed the *Shang Han Lun,* but one of the most significant works to appear was published in the Sung Dynasty. *The Imperial Grace Formulary of the Tai Ping Era,* 1078–1085, became the first codified manual of herb preparations in ancient China.

In the 1800 years since the appearance of Dr. Chang's book, thousands of books have been written in China and Japan that document the clinical work of doctors and their successful treatment of patients. A bibliography of the known works of Oriental Medicine, primarily Chinese, was published in 1819 by the Japanese author Isekiko. It contains references to 2,605 titles of books which appeared between the Han Dynasty (approximately 200 B.C.) and the beginning of the 19th century.

HERBS AND THE FDA

I have included the previous references to show that Western Medicine, or Allopathic medicine as it is sometimes called, is still in its infancy compared to Traditional Chinese Medicine. Western Medicine as we know it came into being in Germany at the end of the 19th Century, a little more than 100 years ago. While there has been much progress and tremendous innovation, Western Medicine is still a young and evolving science.

As the regulatory body of Medicine, the Food and Drug Administration (FDA) is supposed to objectively evaluate and to determine the safety and efficacy of medicines. Unfortunately, the Agency has a bias toward Western Medicine and against herbs, acupuncture, homeopathy, chiropractic, and anything else which could be considered an alternative to Allopathic Medicine. In spite of significant evidence, the FDA continues to dispute the benefits of Herbal Medicine and consequently has placed bureaucratic roadblocks in the way of improving the general health of the United States.

In its entire history, for example, the FDA has never approved an herbal product for any medical use, and only in the past five years has the FDA approved a natural product for its health benefits; it approved basic supplements such as calcium and folic acid only after it was literally compelled to do so by federal legislation.

In contrast, Kommission E, a German Governmental Board, was formed to determine the safety and efficacy of Herbal Medicine. After years of study and careful deliberation, the Kommission found approximately 250 herbs to be safe and effective for medical usage. These herbs, such as ginkgo and milk thistle, were approved only after a thorough review of available research and a study of the safety of each individual herb.

Like Kommission E, the FDA should be proactive in reviewing any treatment which has the potential to be of benefit to human health, instead of standing in the doorway of progress with their collective arms folded, saying "no" to anything that challenges the limits of their understanding.

The FDA's argument is that herbal medicine is unproven, but it is only unproven by their contrived standards. Who decides that the standards of the FDA are the only acceptable standards? Isn't it possible that their prejudices and philosophical blindness may prevent them from being truly objective? Why don't they accept the conclusions of Kommission E?

Sadly, the FDA is more a stone wall than a doorway. Instead of attempting to censor information, the government should be spending its budgetary resources seeking out viable treatments and medicine. By attempting to restrict information and products, the FDA may be doing grave harm to the health of this nation.

DRUGS AND HERBS

The earliest known drug therapy innovation was the smallpox (cowpox) inoculation by Jenner in 1796. Digitalis, a derivative of the herb, foxglove, has probably been in use the longest of any single drug in the Pharmacopoeia of Western Doctors. It has been continuously prescribed for the past 200 years. A popular and well-known medicine like penicillin has been used since 1941, a little more than 50 years.

Currently, pharmaceutical companies develop and patent drugs, selling them until their exclusive patent and high profit margins expire. They then introduce new drugs with high profit margins to replace drugs that have entered the realm of public domain (when anyone can manufacture the drug as a generic and sell it according to more realistic supply and demand cost controls).

Compared to Chinese herbal knowledge and experience, Western pharmaceutical drugs are primarily experimental. While a popular drug like Prozac has been in the marketplace since 1989, and had been studied for perhaps 10 years before its introduction, an herb formula such as Xiao Chai Hu Tang Wan (Minor Bupleurum) first appeared in the *Shang Han Lun* (219 A.D.) and has been in continuous use in China and in the Orient for nearly 2,000 years. If Xiao Chai Hu Tang Wan was one-tenth as dangerous as some drugs on the market today, it would never have survived to the present day.

In this book, there are a number of herb formulas based on the *Shang Han Lun,* which is still the greatest single source of herbal prescriptions in Traditional Chinese Medicine today. In the Sung Dynasty, between the years

982–992, the Chinese Government catalogued all the known herbal medicine of its day and published the renowned compilation, *The Imperial Grace Formulary of the Tai Ping Era*, a book that contains 16,834 entries. A large number of prescriptions from that book are manufactured today. In this book alone, there are at least sixty formulas which appeared in Chinese Medical Literature before the introduction of Jenner's cowpox inoculation at the beginning of the Nineteenth Century.

Chinese Medicine was so far advanced that smallpox inoculation was already widely in use by the sixteenth Century, more than two hundred years before Jenner's supposed discovery. It has been documented that doctors were sent from Turkey and from Czarist Russia to China in 1688 to learn smallpox inoculation from the Chinese.

To further underscore the differences between Traditional Chinese Herbal Medicine and Western Medicine, we should look at the differences in treatment between the two systems. Gastrointestinal (stomach, digestive and intestinal) problems represent the largest block of complaints from patients in the U.S. Yet, Western Medicine offers only three methods of treatment other than surgery. They have anti-ulcer drugs (Tagamet, Zantac), over-the-counter remedies to neutralize stomach acid (Rolaids, Tums, Maalox), and drugs that produce more mucus (Cytotec). These products work by either blocking the production of stomach acid or by producing more mucus in the GI tract to create a barrier which masks the irritation and pain of hydrochloric acid on the stomach lining. Western medicine also offers laxatives to eliminate constipation and antibiotics that stop acute, bacterial diarrhea.

In contrast, Chinese Medicine offers dozens of herbal formulas which enhance the normal function of the digestive system. Instead of blocking symptoms, it concentrates on the root cause so that the symptoms will not reappear. In this book, there are more than twenty-five formulas that directly affect various aspects of digestive function. In Chinese Medicine, there is an entire school of medical thought that links disease to the malfunctioning of digestion. The "Earth Nourishing School" or "Spleen School" evolved in the Sung Dynasty (900–1200 A.D.) and is called the "Earth Nourishing School" because food is derived from the earth and nourishes humankind. It is also called the "Spleen School" because the concept of "spleen" in Chinese Medicine encompasses the digestive functions of the gallbladder, liver, duodenum, pancreas, stomach and spleen.

With more than 2,000 years of experience in treating digestive problems, Traditional Chinese Medicine has developed formulas which improve every aspect of digestion. Four Gentlemen (Si Jun Zi Tang Wan; see page 178) is the foundation for almost all prescriptions which are aimed at tonifying digestion and improving assimilation.

Western Medicine considers many digestive complaints to be psychosomatic. Unfortunately, Western doctors don't have a very sophisticated understanding of some complaints that afflict their patients. There is a tendency when they don't understand a problem to blame their patients by saying "it's all in your head." In other words, there is something mentally wrong with the patient rather than something wrong with the doctor's knowledge.

Problems with digestion are rampant in our society. Evidence of this can be seen in the aisles of supermarkets and drug stores, where shelf after shelf is dedicated to products such as Alka-Seltzer, Milk of Magnesia, and Pepto-Bismol, all of which offer temporary relief from stomach discomfort of one kind or another.

Chinese Herbal Medicine not only provides temporary relief with such products as Pill Curing (traveler's diarrhea, bloating, gas, and discomfort from overeating; see page 230) to treatment of bacterial diarrhea (Huang Lian Su Wan; see pages 165, 235). In between, there are literally dozens of herb formulas to treat and cure digestive problems. With proper diagnosis and the right herb formula, many nagging problems can be eliminated completely or complications can be reduced dramatically.

Chinese Herbal Medicine rarely has the nasty side effects produced by Western pharmaceutical agents, so called sledge-hammer drugs. Herb formulas are often gentle and have a slow but steady, effective rate of improvement.

Herbal treatment for other conditions such as the common cold is vastly superior to the over-the-counter pharmaceuticals available in drugstores and supermarkets. Chinese Medicine recognizes at least several different types of common colds and has developed treatments for each condition and its complications: Common cold with neck pain (Ge Gen Wan); common cold with fever and sore throat (Yin Qiao Jie Du Wan); stomach flu (Huo Xiang Sheng Qi Wan); common cold with alternating chills and fever (Xiao Chai Hu Tang Wan); and common cold with headache (Chuan Xiong Cha Tiao Wan). They also have a 500-year-old formula which strengthens the immune system to prevent the common cold and allergies (Yu Ping Feng San Wan).

In the area of women's menstrual complications, there are very few Western-style treatments except hormone replacement therapy, with its nightmare side effects, and medications like aspirin and Darvon that relieve painful cramping. Traditional Chinese Medicine offers herb formulas to build blood, regulate the menstrual cycle, increase fertility, and stop hot flashes, plus many others.

Another area where Chinese Herbal Medicine is of great benefit is in the nourishing and strengthening of the vital life force energy that wanes as we grow older. Herbal formulas to promote longevity and slow the aging process have been known for centuries in China, beginning with the esoteric practices of Taoist priests in the mountain caves of ancient China.

Modern Chinese Medicine includes formulas which build up that vital life force energy, replenish Qi, and strengthen the kidney energy that is lost in the aging process.

The advantage of Chinese Medicine over Western Medicine is that it offers treatment which promotes the normal function of the body and enhances the organ systems. It can build and strengthen while Western treatment can only cut away offending tissue or attempt to block abnormal function with drugs.

Western drug treatments attack invading pathogens like bacteria (antibiotics) or interfere with the abnormal function of the body (beta-blockers) without treating the cause of disease which is often unknown to modern science. Doctors offer drugs that shrink inflammation (corticosteriods) to temporarily relieve asthma or reduce pain, yet these drugs have debilitating side effects.

The beauty of Chinese Medicine is that there are very few side effects, and herbs can heal with a gentle, lasting efficacy that is recognized by happy patients, not by judgmental government agencies.

WHY CHINESE MEDICINE?

Western doctors treat disease. They are trained in modern medical schools to seek out and eradicate disease. Unfortunately, they know very little about good health. They define good health as the absence of disease. Another drawback to Western treatment is that they seek one single, magic cure, one pill or procedure that will solve the mystery of each disease. This "one-size-fits all" mentality probably comes from their business-oriented outlook. Drug companies look for marketable products. In an attempt to classify and compartmentalize diseases, Western Medicine frequently ignores the individual patient. Researchers want to find the one cure which will help the greatest number of people and make the most money.

Chinese Medicine, on the other hand, treats the patient, not the disease. A doctor of Chinese Medicine studies the patient because people are individuals and each individual is different. Chinese doctors understand that good health is a balance between illness and the individual's constitution. If an individual is truly healthy, then external sickness factors will not cause harm.

This is the real goal of Chinese Medicine: To build strong and healthy human beings. Chinese Herbal Medicine offers people the opportunity to strengthen their immune systems, to improve digestion and to live richer lives.

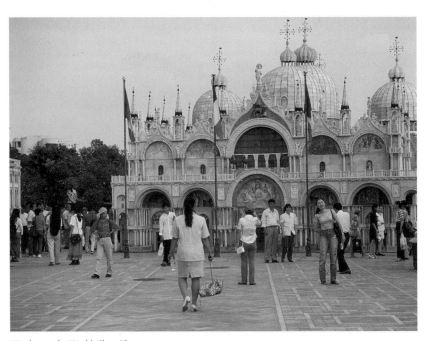

Window to the World, Shen Zhen

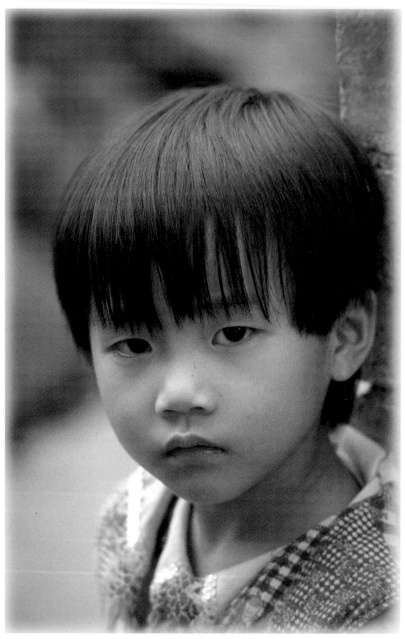

Small child, Guangdong Province

1

TRADITIONAL CHINESE MEDICINE AND MODERN SCIENCE

Traditional Chinese Medicine is often criticized by Western allopathic doctors because it is not "scientifically proven." Much of the resistance of Western-style doctors to Chinese Medicine—and to anything else which could be considered an alternative to Western-style medicine—comes from doctors who claim that TCM and other modalities haven't been studied by the same standards of proof as American medicines.

We see this argument echoed every day in the popular press: "Where's the proof?" asks Dr. John Weiler in the May 12, 1997, issue of *Time* magazine. "If you have something novel, you have an obligation to show your studies."[1] It is assumed by Dr. Weiler and by many others in the medical/scientific community that studies are the only way to validate medicine. In their opinion, any form of medicine is invalid without studies. These studies are supposedly unbiased and accurate demonstrations of the scientific method which show no cultural or economic bias. They are meant to substantiate the efficacy of medicine. It is also assumed that all Western-style medicine available today has been carefully and fairly evaluated, so that anything introduced in the future is, as Dr. Weiler puts it, "novel."

What is this supposed scientific method? The recognition of a problem (in the case of medicine, a disease), a hypothesis of cause (diagnosis), the prediction of a solution (a possible cure), experiments to test the hypothesis and solution (a treatment protocol) and simple rules that organize the entire process. This again is the "one-size-fits-all" mentality of Western Medicine. Simply put, Western doctors aspire to treat all diseases of the same name (asthma; diabetes; eczema) with exactly the same treatment.

The FDA requires this demonstration of evidence in order to approve drugs for use in this country. Animal studies are required to demonstrate safety before human tests can be conducted. All of this evidence, double-blind studies, control groups and placebos are necessary in order to assess the safety and efficacy of any medicine, according to protocols established by the FDA.

The cost of such studies is enormous, of course, ranging between $100 million and $250 million per drug ingredient. The major drug companies fund most of the studies in the hope that their research will yield valuable and effective medicines from which they can recoup their investment. "If they were to recover the massive investment all this involved, they would first have to secure a patent for their drug and so make sure of cornering the market; secondly, they needed to be sure the market was as big as possible."[2]

It is then argued that Chinese Medicine and anything else which is "novel" or different from the norm hasn't followed these rules and is therefore considered invalid. Until Chinese Medicine is judged by the same standards and methodology as medicines produced by American pharmaceutical companies, it will remain invalid. This argument is commonly used by state governments and the FDA to ban alternative treatments and alternative products. State and federal agencies contend that it is merely anecdotal evidence that some substances such as herbs may have been used in other countries for hundreds, if not thousands of years. They categorize this as "folk" medicine. According to these government agencies, a history of long-term use does not prove that herbs are harmless or that they have any real value. Government logic is that "unproven remedies" may keep people from using "scientifically proven treatments," and taking "folk" remedies may delay a sick individual from seeking proper medical care.

"There is also much to be lost if we drift from our scientific moorings and allow the marketplace to be filled with unsupported claims on products of unproven safety," asserted Michael Taylor, deputy commissioner of the FDA in 1993.[3] "The public's health could be at risk, proven therapies and interventions may be passed up, and scarce health-care dollars will be wasted."

This attitude about the scientific method contains a variety of assumptions. The first assumption is that human beings and their conditions or diseases can be understood, quantified, or measured with technological equipment. Next, it assumes that it is possible to measure diseases and disease conditions. Finally, it assumes that the modern world has the sophistication and the scientific instruments to accurately do the measuring. For a "science" that is barely 100 years old, these assumptions are rather bold.

In this day and age, when a "new" disease like Chronic Fatigue Syndrome is discovered, it is given a name and investigations are begun, directed toward finding a treatment. An assumption is made that all people who manifest a disease can be given the same treatment and that a cure will follow. If the hypothesis is correct and the treatment follows according to plan, then the solution is undeniable and has been proven scientifically.

Unfortunately, human beings are incredibly complex. They do not always fit neatly into protocols and studies. Traditional Chinese Medicine approaches each patient as a unique individual. It examines each person individually to determine how they are similar or dissimilar to other patients with the same symptoms. Instead of looking for new cures and new treatments, classical Chinese doctors looked to the past to discern the pattern of disease. They chose to learn from the experiences of doctors who had gone before them. Patterns of human disease have been studied in China since before recorded history; a body of knowledge has been accumulated for more than 2,000 years. In 220 B.C., some of this accumulated knowledge was collected and published in the *Yellow Emperor's Classic of Medicine*. This text advised that a dedicated doctor should study the classics—the volumes of books written before 200 B.C. "This is recorded in the ancient books,"[4] which hold the key to understanding the healing of the human condition. Even 2,000 years ago, it was recognized that many of the answers to healthcare were well known, and that there was already an established body of knowledge available to the practitioner. This knowledge has been passed down through the last two millennia from doctor to apprentice and, in more recent times, through a university education.

When Chinese Medicine was in its infancy, there were no books, no scientific instruments, no quantitative tests nor extensive, gleaming laboratories. As a consequence, Chinese Medicine developed in a manner in which laboratory tests were unnecessary. Much of that testing remains unnecessary today. Certain procedures were followed, but they were not the same procedures as those which evolved in the labs and hospitals of Western medicine.

In judging any medicine, a number of assumptions come into play. The first assumption is that Western Medicine is scientifically proven. This alone is in great dispute. "The great secret, known to internists…but still hidden from the general public, is that most things get better by themselves. Most things, in fact, are better by the morning."[5] It is commonly assumed that modern medicines available in America are tested and judged "scientifically"—when in reality more than 70% of all modern medicines are not scientifically proven. "The National Academy of Sciences-National Research Council…reviewed all prescription drugs marketed between 1938 and 1962 to determine if they complied with the 1962 drug amendments…The FDA also conducted a major investigation which confirmed that thousands of drugs lacked evidence of effectiveness."[6] Many of those drugs remain in the marketplace today. Accordingly, there are literally thousands of drugs which have proven to be ineffective, yet doctors continue to prescribe them to their patients because they believe them to be useful even if scientific studies prove them to be useless and possibly dangerous.[7]

"People have always tended to adopt general rules, beliefs, creeds, ideas, and hypotheses without thoroughly questioning their validity and to retain them long after they have been shown to be meaningless, false or at least questionable. The most widespread assumptions are often the least questioned."[8] Doctors are no exception to this rule. "Scientists must accept their experimental findings even when they would like them to be different. They must strive to distinguish between what they see and what they wish to see."[9]

In fact, it is common practice among doctors to develop experimental treatments without having any idea whether the procedures they attempt will be of benefit: "In the United States, coronary artery bypass surgery was widely adopted before any studies had shown it to be effective in preventing death or disability."[10] Medical doctors in this country frequently experiment, quickly adopting new or innovative treatments in order to improve their patient's care. "Coronary bypass surgery caught on very quickly in the United States, reaching rates up to 28 times that in some European countries."[11] These statistics also apply to many different surgical procedures, the rates of which dwarf those in Europe. In the U.S., for example, "one study found three times as many mastectomies in New England as in England or Sweden, even though the rate of breast cancer was similar."[12]

There is another even more significant illusion. It is that all medicines can be tested and proven according to the protocol of modern science. "Modern Western-style medicine and pharmacy are the only therapeutic systems that base large parts of their knowledge and practice on technical criteria, thus allowing for a high degree of standardization both of therapeutic procedures and of the means employed in therapy."[13] In short, the testing of modern drug-like substances in laboratories generally applies only to pharmaceutical, Western-style medicines. Any attempt to judge other modalities of treatment, such as homeopathy, cannot be proven by the standards of modern science. "No therapeutic system outside of modern scientific medicine can be completely legitimized by scientific principles."[14]

Another popular illusion about medicine, especially so-called modern Western-style medicine, is that it is practiced in every corner of the globe. This is, in fact, not the case. In France, Great Britain, and Germany, on which the North American model was based, the practice of medicine is very different. "How can medicine, which is commonly supposed to be a science, particularly in the United States, be so different in four countries whose people are so similar genetically? The answer is that while medicine benefits from a certain amount of scientific input, culture intervenes at every step of the way."[15]

"One World Health Organization study found that doctors from different countries diagnosed different causes of death even when shown identical information from the same death certificate."[16] How can this be? In a scientific world, all answers should be the same because the data is objective and clear. Unfortunately, data is one issue, but the analysis of that data is another. So the illusion is that medicine, especially in the U.S., is scientifically based and objective. Doctors are expected to follow identical "standards of practice."

Cultural bias seems to play a big part in medicine. Coronary bypass surgery is very popular among Western-style doctors because it mirrors our own culture: "The popularity of coronary bypass surgery concords with the American culture biases of aggressive treatment and with the American view of the body as a machine."[17] Diseases are categorized, summarized and systematized; protocols are established. Internal organs are replaced like engine parts because some American doctors feel they are unnecessary. According to *Novak's Textbook of Gynecology:* "Menstruation is a nuisance to most women, and if this can be abolished without impairing ovarian function, it would probably be a blessing to not only the woman but her husband."[18] Because many doctors are men and modern medicine is dominated by males, women are afforded little respect or compassion: "After the last planned pregnancy, the uterus becomes a useless, bleeding, symptom-producing, potentially cancer-bearing organ and therefore should be removed."[19] The arrogance of modern American medicine takes many forms and reflects an insensitivity to patients, as well as an abhorrence of nature and the natural world. In contrast, French Doctors seem to try much harder to keep women whole: "comparisons have shown that the proportion of hysterectomized women in France is lower than that in England, and the English hysterectomy rate is not even half the U.S. rate."[20]

"If we don't describe it first, our first reaction is always negative. We are very chauvinistic and have the attitude that if we haven't found something, it's probably wrong," states one American doctor.[21] "The American public does not have the knowledge to make wise healthcare decisions," states Dr. David Kessler, former FDA Commissioner. "FDA is the arbiter of truth. Trust us. We will tell you what's good for you."[22]

Consequently, when something as different as Chinese Medicine is presented to Western doctors, their reaction is often immediate rejection. Although Chinese Medicine has been practiced for more than three millennia and is the primary healthcare system for the majority of the population of the world today, it is still not fully accepted in this country. Why?

The scope of practice of Chinese Medicine is very limited in U.S. states where acupuncture is legal. Many diseases are not legally treatable by acupuncture and herbalism—even though there are extremely effective and widely used remedies available. Acupuncture, according to the law of the State of California, can be used only "to prevent or modify the perception of pain or to normalize physiological functions, including pain control, for the treatment of certain diseases or dysfunctions of the body."[23] There is ample proof of the effectiveness of Traditional Chinese Medicine; thousands of studies exist. But, unfortunately, most of them are written in Chinese and haven't been translated into English. This does not seem to positively influence the judgment of government.

As an example of medical prejudice, 21 states do not recognize acupuncture as a viable medicine. North Dakota is one such state: "The practice of acupuncture has not been recognized by the Legislative Assembly of North Dakota as a distinct healing art."[24] Thirteen states do not offer acupuncturists a license, yet these same states permit medical doctors to practice acupuncture without any specific training or experience. Until 1996, the FDA classified the acupuncture needle as an "experimental medical device" even though acupuncture needles have been used since before recorded history. "According to *Shi Ji (Records of the Historian)* written in 104–91 B.C., the celebrated physician Bian Que, who lived in the 5th century B.C., successfully employed diagnostic pulse feeling and acupuncture treatment."[25]

"Most often, when an idea is adopted, particular attention is given to cases that seem to support it, while cases that seem to refute it are distorted, belittled, or ignored," writes scientist Paul Hewitt. "Scientists, like most people, have a vast capacity for fooling themselves."[26]

"There's no evidence," says Dr. Graham Woolf, a gastroenterologist at UCLA-Cedars-Sinai Medical Center, "that garlic does anything but make your breath smell."[27] Garlic (Da Suan in Chinese) has been studied both here and in China. "To our astonishment, we found that some 700 papers had been published over the last 20 years."[28] These hundreds of studies have demonstrated that garlic is effective in treating many different disease conditions.[29] In addition to its effectiveness in expelling parasites which was documented in the 5th century A.D. Chinese publication, *Collection of Commentaries on the Classic of the Materia Medica,*[30] garlic has been shown to be 88% effective in treating amoebic dysentery in modern clinical trials. It has also been effective in treating pinworms, has been proven to kill Staphylococcus aureus, Streptococcus pneumoniae, Neisseria meningitis, Salmonella typhi, and Corynebacterium diphtheriae bacteria. Garlic has antifungal properties, acts as an antibiotic and is anti-neoplastic (anti-cancer),[31] all of which have been demonstrated in animal and human studies.

Another very popular Western herb, Echinacea, has been widely studied in Germany, the leading country in developing modern phyto-medicines (medicines derived from plants). Echinacea's effectiveness as a non-specific immune enhancer has been carefully and scientifically documented for more than 50 years. "From 1940 through the present time, there have been over 200 papers published on the chemistry, pharmacology and clinical applications" of Echinacea.[32] "German researchers have performed most of the studies."[33] In fact, while the study of the value of herbs has been going on in Germany for decades, the FDA refuses to recognize any medicinal value in herbs and has never approved an herbal product for the treatment of any disease. "Kommission E in Germany (the German FDA) has prepared nearly 300 monographs on medicinal plants"[34] regarding their accepted medicinal uses.

"Echinacea was not introduced under authoritative auspices…On the contrary, its origin as a constituent of a 'home cure' remedy made by an illiterate, unknown physician, was used as an argument to authoritatively condemn it."[35]

And why aren't more studies performed in the U.S? Why aren't studies from other countries accepted? Is this the only country in the world in which science is practiced? "Much medical research these days is funded by the pharmaceutical industry, and here there is always a certain amount of pressure to find results that will be favorable to the drug the company sells."[36] Could this then explain why the medical world might not be receptive to herbal medicine which cannot be patented? "Richard A Davidson, M.D., an associate professor in the Department of Medicine at the University of Florida in Gainesville, found that studies supported by pharmaceutical companies were much more likely to find new therapies superior to old than were studies that apparently didn't receive funds from the pharmaceutical industry."[37]

And what is the value of these studies anyway? It was acknowledged in Time magazine that "Doctors note that in trials of new drugs, as many as 20% to 40% of the participants improve even if they have got nothing more than sugar water."[38] Are these supposed "scientific studies" truly science, or are they just the patina of science? Is it not a concern that the very people doing the testing on supposedly scientifically-proven medicine are the same people who stand to benefit economically from their FDA approval? Isn't it odd that the same people who stand to lose the most to possible competition are the same ones who attack the alternatives? "When an idea is adopted, particular attention is given to cases that seem to support it, while cases that seem to refute it are distorted, belittled, or ignored."[39]

For example, several years ago the FDA reviewed a study of the herb, saw palmetto (serenoa repens). Saw palmetto has been widely used in France as the over-the-counter treatment of choice by millions of French men for Benign Prostate Hypertrophy. Although the study followed FDA protocol and resulted in "statistically significant improvements," in review the FDA refused to permit a health claim for this product.[40] Why? In the Federal Register, the FDA wrote: "Although the Champault study suggests that patients treated with PA 109 (saw palmetto extract) showed some statistical improvements in symptoms associated with benign prostatic hypertrophy, the results are not considered clinically significant, i.e., the symptoms continue to exist and the patient is not medically better."[41] In other words, the patients improved considerably, but some effects of an enlarged prostate still remained. What was the FDA's justification for this decision? "As long as only the symptoms of the condition are relieved, individuals who fear surgery may be lulled into a false sense of security and thus delay reexamination by a physician, resulting in a delay in treatment of the disease."[42] Only a few months following this decision, the FDA approved Proscar, a drug with similar qualities to saw palmetto.

How far will medical people go in attacking alternatives to the "standards of practice" in America? In a court case regarding chelation therapy, Dr. Warren

Levin was charged with "unprofessional conduct" by the New York State Medical Board—even though chelation therapy is legal in New York. One expert witness, Dr. Michael Herman, testified under oath that chelation therapy was "worthless" and no "good" cardiologist would use it. Under cross-examination, Dr. Herman testified that chelation therapy was never offered as a course at any time during his medical education, nor was it even considered as a treatment during his fellowship at Harvard. He testified that he had personally never spoken with a doctor who had used it. He also testified that he had not read any of the other testimony regarding the benefits of chelation therapy and had not done a computer search of any literature seeking any information on chelation therapy. He therefore knew nothing about the specific subject about which he was testifying as an "expert" witness in a medical ethics case.

It is evident that viable and effective treatments of some diseases may be impeded by the staunch attacks of those who through ignorance or malice would slander alternatives which they either don't understand or don't want to understand. This is painfully obvious in the area of cancer treatment in particular because the treatment of cancer is the most legally proscribed of all treatment protocols: "Out here in the trenches we are absolutely gagged with government regulations of all kinds," writes Dr. Francis M. Powers, of Cancer Treatment Associates in Williamsport, PA.[43] Anyone offering unconventional alternatives to chemotherapy and surgery are attacked unmercifully by the authorities. But, modern research in China has demonstrated that herbal treatments are more effective than conventional treatments and have fewer negative side effects.[44] Doctors in China often give their patients the classic herb formula Four Gentlemen which consists of four herbs to improve digestion. This herb formula first appeared in Chinese medical literature in the *Imperial Grace Formulary of the Tai Ping Era* which was issued by the Imperial Medical Department of the Sung Dynasty between 1078–1085.[45] Modern research in China has shown that in combination with chemotherapy and radiation, it protects normal cells, reduces the side effects of chemotherapy, helps the body resist bone marrow suppression, helps maintain the counts of red blood cells and white blood cells at normal levels, stops cancer cells from rebounding and inhibits metastasization.[46]

"In the People's Republic a large number of research institutes have been established where clinical and theoretical issues of Traditional Chinese Medicine are studied."[47] Among the results of this research was the publication of a *Comprehensive Dictionary of Chinese Pharmaceutics* which was published by the Shanghai People's Press in 1977. It lists "5,767 monographs on items used as drugs (natural substances, plant, animal and mineral) in Traditional Chinese pharmacy."[48]

In studies done at Beijing Chinese Japanese Friendship Hospital and the Shanghai TCM University Long Hua Hospital, patients with advanced cases of non-surgically treatable liver cancer given only herbs had a three year survival rate of 37.72%; a group given only chemotherapy had a three year survival rate of 7.62%.[49] In another study of advanced lung cancer, the two year survival rate with herbal treatment was 13.3% while the chemotherapy rate was 3.3%.[50] In still another study, stage three liver cancer patients given only herbal treatment had a 20% survival rate after 12 months while the chemotherapy group had no survivors after 12 months.[51] Finally, another study at the Tumor Hospital at Shanghai Medical University, 228 advanced liver cancer cases were studied from 1981–1990. The first group was given radiation treatment plus Four Gentlemen herb formula while the second group was treated with radiation alone. The five year survival rate for the combined group was 42.97% with a mean survival time of 53.4 months while the group that received radiation alone had a five year survival rate of 14.48% with a mean survival time of 11.1 months.[52] These are long-term studies, some that included as many as 996 patients, whose cases were followed carefully for several years.

"As American medical education became increasingly dominated by scientists and researchers, doctors came to be trained according to the values and standards of academic specialists. Many have argued that this was a mistake."[53] It has been considered a mistake because modern medicine has lost touch with its patients; it seems to be caught up in laboratory science rather than providing relief to human beings who are ill. "A patient seeing a general practitioner (GP) here in the U.S. will have more tests than would the patient seeing the GP in practically any European country."[54] And what is the value of these tests? Are they really valuable? Do they prove anything? "Diagnostic testing is largely unregulated, even at the elementary level of ensuring that equipment is accurate and that trained people are reading the test results under optimal conditions."[55]

"A person who is restricted to laboratory experiments, especially if he be more or less adversely prejudiced...is not in a position to judge with discretion. Nor is a laboratory man to be considered an 'authority' in clinical directions," wrote John Lloyd, past president of the American Pharmaceutical Association.[56]

It is especially dangerous and detrimental to the health of every individual in the country if legislative decisions continue to be based on the views of laboratory results rather than clinical experience with actual human patients. It could lead to a restriction of our freedom of choice and cause progress in treating patients to cease. There is no single, perfect system of medicine which should exclude all others. What we should seek out is "therapeutic plurality" in "unstructured coexistence" among all forms of medicine. In other words, the marketplace should determine the availability of products; the consumer should have the freedom to choose his or her own form of treatment. Otherwise, "the only alternative would be a repressive policy where the viewpoints of one group in society are enforced as the standards of the entire population."[57]

In the case of Chinese Medicine, centuries of knowledge and experience in treating patients has been ignored by the FDA because of an obvious bias against herbal medicine. The chemical complexity of herbs does not fit neatly into the laboratory experiments demanded of them by officials of the FDA. "Nutrition and nutritional therapies are an evolving science with no one having any corner on the knowledge," writes Dr. Powers. "To think the FDA can even appreciate the subtleties is ridiculous."[58]

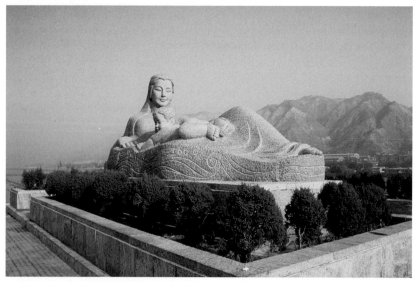

Goddess of the Yellow River, Lanzhou

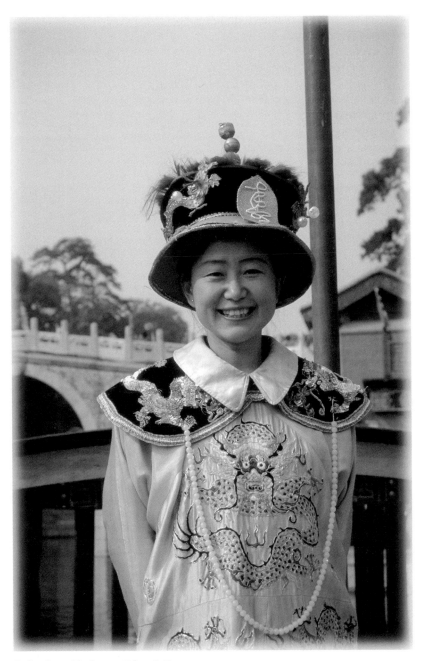

Suzhou Street, The Summer Palace, Beijing

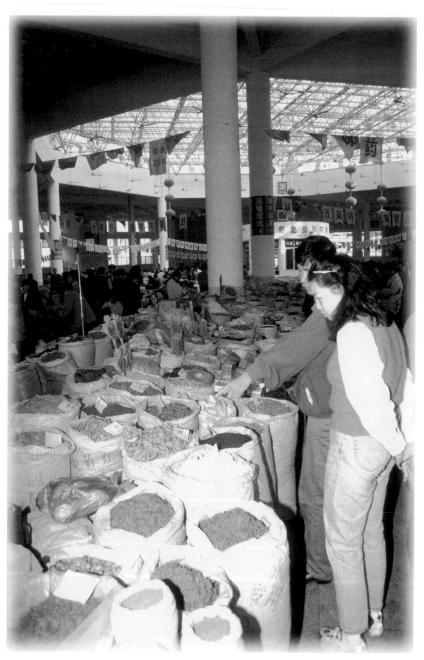

Herb Farmer's Market, Anguo

2

COUNTERFEITING AND MOUNTAIN BANDIT FACTORIES

For years, tourists could buy a fake Rolex watch on the streets of Hong Kong for a fraction of the price of a real Rolex. Fake audio tapes, videos, software, cameras, CD players, and designer clothing used to be easily acquired on the streets and in the shops of Hong Kong, but counterfeiting has not been limited to that city. It is rampant throughout Asia. Because of widespread counterfeiting in China, for example, the United States government has been trying to enforce patent and copyright laws for many years in an effort to stop piracy and the counterfeiting of American products like computer software.

What does this have to do with Chinese herbal products? In China, there are counterfeiters of herbal products as well as counterfeiters of software and video tapes. Many popular herbal products are copied and sold in herb shops from Beijing to Guangzhou, and a good many of these fake products are smuggled into the United States. Here, they can be purchased by a public which, for the most part, is completely unaware of the differences between legitimate herb products and fakes.

It has been estimated that 70% of the patent medicines sold in Chinese herb shops in the U.S. are smuggled and/or counterfeit. My own observations in various American Chinatown herb shops support this claim. Having visited Chinese herb shops all over mainland China, Singapore, Hong Kong, Thailand, Indonesia and Malaysia, as well as in New York, Oakland, San Francisco, San Jose and Los Angeles, I have observed a large number of smuggled, illegal products of dubious medicinal value. Speaking from experience, it is very difficult to distinguish a legitimate product from a fake. Only a trained observer with significant experience can make these distinctions.

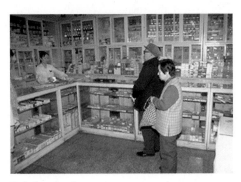

Herb shop, Lanzhou

Where do these products come from? Who makes them? Why do they exist? In China, they call counterfeit factories "Mountain Bandit Factories" or "mountainside factories." The idea comes from a lawless time when bandits hid in the mountains and preyed on innocent travelers. These bogus factories often have no license, have not been inspected, and make product which is inferior to the medicine produced in legitimate, high-quality factories. A mountain bandit factory will produce an herb formula and copy the packaging in order to capitalize on the reputation of the best factories.

Mountain Bandit Factories do not have quality control standards established by the government. Who knows if they even have quality control standards? No one inspects these factories to determine whether they adhere to health, sanitation, and safety codes or whether they follow any standards in the production of these fake products. They often add illegal pharmaceutical drugs to products in order to get quick, dramatic results. At best, they cut corners in their production process in order to lower costs and produce a cheaper product. They are not inspected to ensure that they follow any standards of cleanliness.

In China, the poorest quality herbs are processed and dried in the street. (Please see the photos below.) In all probability, low-quality herbs like these end up in counterfeit medicines in order to cut costs.

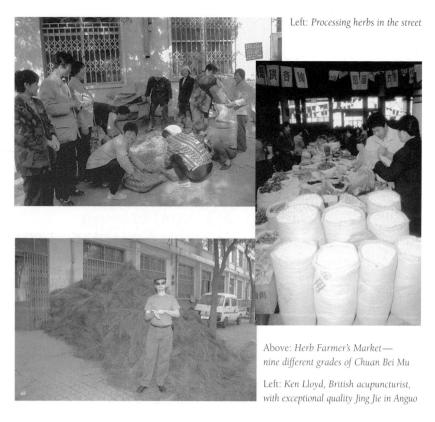

Left: *Processing herbs in the street*

Above: *Herb Farmer's Market—*
nine different grades of Chuan Bei Mu

Left: *Ken Lloyd, British acupuncturist,*
with exceptional quality Jing Jie in Anguo

As a National Board Certified Chinese herbalist, I have visited China a number of times to familiarize myself with the Chinese herb world. On the occasion of the photos below, I was in the company of Ken Lloyd, a licensed Acupuncturist and Chinese Herbalist from England. We spent an afternoon trying to identify herbs that we found being processed on the sidewalks. Our general conclusion was that most of these herbs were of inferior quality and the standards of processing left a great deal to be desired.

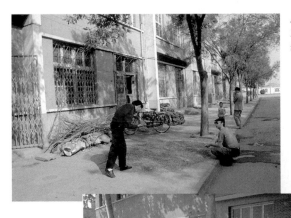

All photos this page:
*Ken Lloyd examining herbs
in streets of Anguo*

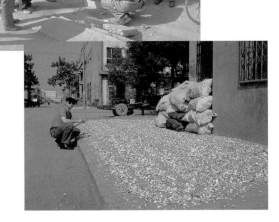

Who buys these herbs? Where do they end up? I know that they are not found in the medicines manufactured by licensed factories. I have inspected the raw materials stored in the warehouses of International GMP certified factories (see *What Is GMP?* page 51), and the herbs they use are high quality. In fact, I was surprised by the high quality of herbs that I saw in GMP factories. The herbs are equal to the best grades of herbs that I have seen in the most expensive herb shops in the U.S.

Unfortunately, it is impossible to determine the quality of herbs found in Patent Medicines without expensive testing, and even with testing it is difficult to identify the quality of individual herbs, once they have been cooked together. The only way to be assured of quality is by inspecting the production facilities, examining the samples of raw materials used in manufacture, and visiting the sources of those raw materials.

In my visits to China, I have walked in the fields, visited the processing centers of raw herbs, and toured the best factories in order to understand where to get the best products.

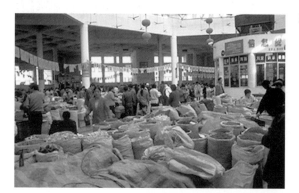

Herb Farmer's Market, Anguo

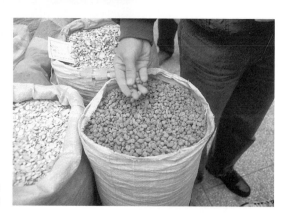

Yan Hu Suo (corydalis) in Farmer's Market

Independent tests of counterfeit products have detected extremely high heavy metal content (lead, mercury and arsenic) which would never be allowed in legal products. Some counterfeit products may contain only fillers such as cornstarch, illegal pharmaceutical drugs, and synthetic colors. It is rare to see illegal ingredients listed on the packaging, but it does happen on occasion.

Below, I have included photographs of products in order to show how difficult it might be for the unsuspecting shopper to distinguish between quality products and counterfeits. Please note the different packaging on four different boxes of Pill Curing, a formula used for treating upset stomach.

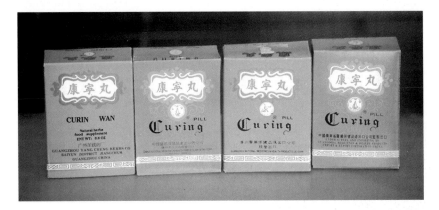

These appear to be the same product, but each one is manufactured by a different factory. How can one determine which is the legitimate product? Sometimes, it is very difficult. Inside, one may find that the size of the pills will vary or the color may be different. Please notice different logos on three of the boxes. Also notice that three of the packages are Yang Cheng Brand while the fourth is Wu Yang Brand. Yang Cheng Brand is the label for an import/export company from southern China; this company, I have been told, contracts the manufacturing of this product from different factories while selling it under their own label. I haven't visited any of the factories and I cannot vouch for their quality.

Please see photo below of seven bottles of Pe Min Kan Wan, a formula used for allergies and sinus congestion. Which one is produced by the legitimate manufacturer? The boxes have different logos and different brand names, but they look alike. One bottle simply states that it is "Made in the People's Republic of China." There is no indication where it was manufactured or which company produced it. It was simply made somewhere in China.

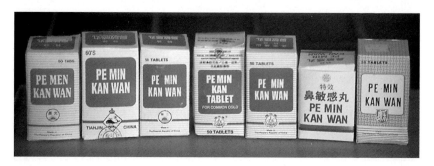

Some samples of Pe Min Kan Wan have been tested and have been found to contain three different pharmaceutical drugs (chlorpheniramine maleate, acetaminophen, phenylpropanolamine hydrochloride) as well as synthetic food coloring (FD & C #5 and FD & C #1). Usually, these drugs are not listed on the labels and are therefore being consumed by an unsuspecting public.

Because Pe Min Kan Wan has a reputation for being a very effective treatment for sinus congestion and allergies which are common problems here in the U.S., it has become well known outside the Chinese community. I have seen counterfeit versions of Pe Min Kan Wan in health food stores, grocery markets and convenience stores, as well as in the offices of licensed acupuncturists.

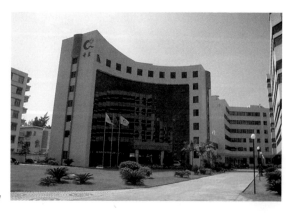

Guangzhou Qi Xing Factory

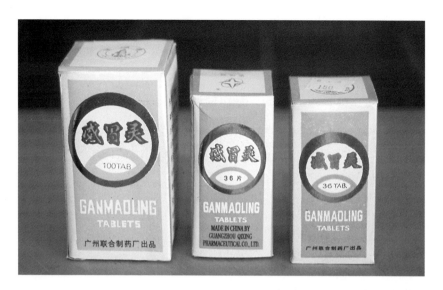

Gan Mao Ling, a popular common cold medicine, is another example of a high-quality product which is being counterfeited and sold in the U.S. The photo above shows three bottles of Gan Mao Ling, two of which have been tested and have been found to contain three drugs (acetaminophen, chlorpheniramine maleate, and caffeine) as well as synthetic food coloring. The Chinese characters on two of the boxes read Guangzhou United Pharmaceutical Factory. It is my understanding that there is no such factory. (One sure tip off that a product is smuggled is that it has only Chinese characters on the label; in order to be legally imported into the U.S., a product must have English lettering noting where it was made as well as other requirements.) Who knows where these factories are located? Who knows what quality of product they manufacture? Are they licensed or inspected?

The middle bottle in the above photograph is made by an International GMP certified manufacturer—the Guangzhou Qi Xing Pharmaceutical Company. I visited this factory in October 1996 and in October 1997 (see photo, opposing page). I do not have pictures inside the production facilities because they did not allow me to take photos in the factory itself, but I was satisfied by my inspection. The Gan Mao Ling in the photograph, however, contains synthetic yellow dye and therefore I cannot recommend it. I prefer Plum Flower Brand Gan Mao Ling, because it is produced by this factory, but it does not contain yellow dye.

As I have said, it is difficult to tell which product is legitimate. For example, on the following page is a photo of three bottles of Kang Gu Zeng Sheng Pian. The packaging of each bottle is distinct; the bottles themselves are quite different: one is glass, two are plastic. Each label is different. One bottle is Fen Kiang Brand, a second bottle is Chu Kiang Brand, while the third lists no brand name. How can anyone be expected to tell the difference between them? Which one is the real product?

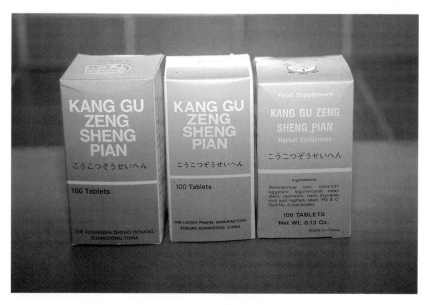

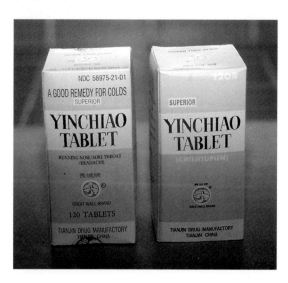

In the next photo, two bottles of Yin Chiao Chieh Tu Pien are shown. One bottle is plain and makes no claims, while the other bottle states that it is "a good remedy for colds," and is good for treating "running nose / sore throat / and headache" (sic). They both appear to be made in the same factory, but they are not the same. The bottle with the claims also lists drugs contained in the tablets: acetaminophen and chlorpheniramine maleate. Other versions of Yin Chiao have been tested in independent laboratories and have also been found to contain synthetic drugs. Again, I recommend Plum Flower Brand Yin Qiao because it contains no drugs or food colorings.

As I have mentioned, some Chinese patent medicines have been tested and have been found to contain illegal pharmaceutical drugs as well as synthetic food coloring. Who knows what else they contain? "The presence of drugs in Chinese herbal products ("patent medicines") was first revealed in two items among the many U.S. imports of the 1980's."[59]

Counterfeiting is a major problem because bogus products financially harm the reputation and the brand name of legitimate manufacturers who follow strict quality controls and produce high-quality products. It is far more expensive to produce legitimate, high-quality products than to produce fakes. Fakes are smuggled into other countries, bypassing quality standards and inspections. Manufacturers of these bogus products exploit unsuspecting, uninformed consumers who may be suckered into paying a little less for a product which is inferior. Patients in clinics are harmed because their conditions do not improve as they should, and the reputation of Chinese Medicine is damaged because people don't get positive results. Unhappy patients blame doctors, herbs, or Chinese Medicine itself for not being effective.

The photo to the right is of a sign hanging in a TCM hospital in Beijing. The sign warns patients against the unscrupulous manufacturers of bogus, counterfeit medicines.

It would be very tempting for an unlicensed factory in China to cut corners by using poor quality herbs in their products. Once they are manufactured, it is much more difficult to determine the quality of the herbal ingredi-

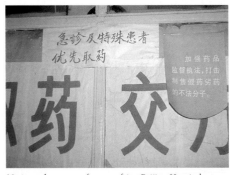

Notice to be aware of counterfeits, Beijing Hospital

ents inside. In China, there are many different grades of herbs, and while the best factories use very high-quality herbs in their products, mountain bandit factories or factories of lesser integrity may use herbs literally bought off the street.

The only way to protect yourself and your family from low-quality products is purchase known high-quality products from legitimate manufacturers. High-quality manufacturers use top grade herbs which have been handled with great care.

Unfortunately, in both the U.S. and in China, the only way to know for certain you are buying quality products is to find a reliable source. Right now, there are only a few companies who are working to ensure quality. Personally, I recommend Plum Flower Brand Products produced by Mayway Corporation in Oakland, California. I have visited their raw herb processing facilities in China

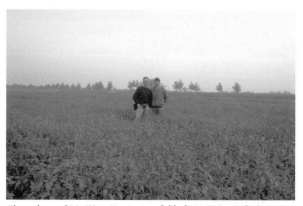

and walked in the herb fields with their Chinese representatives to follow their handling of herbal products from the field to the package.

Mayway's house label, Plum Flower Brand, has one distinct advantage over all other Chinese products: there are no counterfeits. You

The author and Mr. Wang Yun-Jin in a field of Niu Xi (acyanthes), Anguo

can be assured that you are getting the best. All products available under the Plum Flower Brand are high-quality Chinese herb products that are tested in independent labs and are guaranteed to be drug-free. Factories producing herbal medicines sold under the Plum Flower Classics Brand are International GMP certified. See *What Is GMP?* page 51.

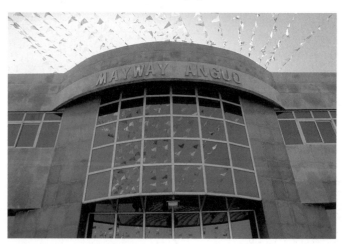

Mayway Anguo herb processing

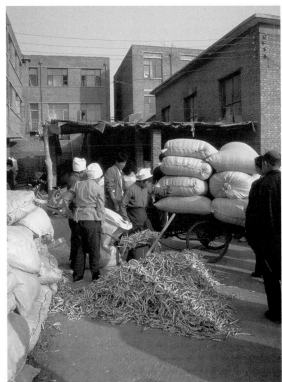

Photos this page:
*Herb wholesale market,
Anguo*

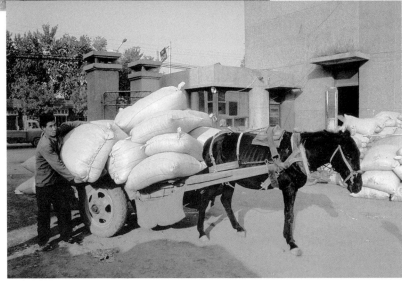

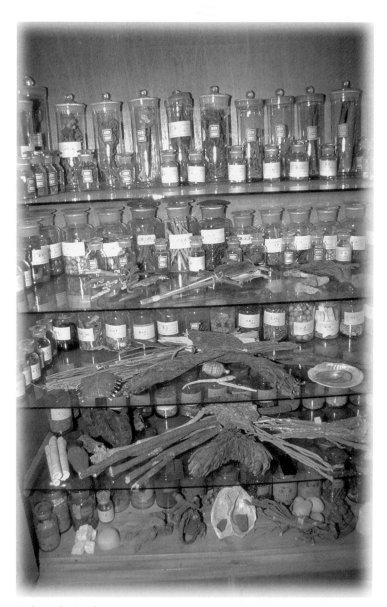

Herb samples, Lanzhou

3

LANZHOU FOCI HERB FACTORY

In my travels to China, I have had the opportunity to visit several manufacturing facilities in various parts of that country. I have also visited a variety of manufacturing facilities in the U.S. which are producing Chinese herbal products, more traditional vitamins, and Western herbal products. It is my opinion that the manufacturing and production quality of the best Chinese factories is superior to most of their counterparts in the U.S. They are equal to the very best manufacturers in the world.

I have chosen to give the Lanzhou Foci herb company products a prominent place in this book because they have a large selection of the highest quality products available. I highly recommend Lanzhou Foci herb products because, to my knowledge, they are among the best available in the world. I take them personally and recommend them to my patients.

THE HISTORY OF LANZHOU FOCI HERB FACTORY

The Lanzhou Foci Herb Factory was established in Shanghai in 1929 to produce traditional herb formulas in pill form utilizing modern technology. As such, it was the first factory in China to apply new technology to the production of classic herbal pill formulas. Following the successful introduction of what have come to be called "patent medicines," the factory began to export their pill formulas in 1930 to Malaysia and Hong Kong.

It was the original intention of the factory's founders to produce high-quality, easy-to-swallow, small pills which would last a long time preserved in glass bottles, and to produce the time-tested herb formulas published in classic herb books such as the *Shang Han Lun*.

The original Lanzhou commitment to produce classic traditional herb formulas using modern, state-of-the-art technological methods is followed today at the current factory which moved to Lanzhou, Giansu Province, in 1956. The factory was relocated because the new area's dry climate and clean environment made it possible to produce the highest quality products and because of the wide availability of high-quality herbs, especially tonic herbs, in nearby agricultural fields.

The Lanzhou Foci factory has always had a reputation for producing the best herbal pill products in China. For many years, it was considered to be the number one ranked factory in China. In order to maintain that reputation, the Lanzhou factory began to build newly upgraded facilities in 1994. Completion of the new factory occurred on November 18, 1996, and they were certified a

"Good Manufacturing Practices" factory in August of 1996 after an inspection by the Australian Therapeutic Goods Administration, which is widely reputed to have the highest standards of certification in the world. Such a certification is highly prized in China. At present, there are probably no more than 10 factories with equal certification.

LANZHOU FOCI PHARMACEUTICAL FACTORY QUALITY CONTROL

1. The fields are physically inspected to ensure that the herbs are grown in accordance to rigid standards, using no chemicals or pesticides in the growing process. The herbs are not certified organic because Lanzhou has never participated in a third party certification program, but the factory's own tests indicate that there are almost no pesticide residues in their raw herbs or finished products. A sample of each batch of raw herbs is stored with a lot number, purchase date and source.
2. The factory moved to Lanzhou in order to capitalize on the dry climate which is especially important in the preservation of herbs. The dry climate makes it possible to avoid using chemicals, such as preservatives like sulfur and chlorine, in the manufacturing process.
3. They inspect and analyze all herbs before they enter the warehouse for quality, size, smell, taste and active ingredients. They test to identify the herb's unique chemical structure or "fingerprint." They also test for heavy metals, such as lead, mercury and arsenic, as well for molds and yeast. Tests for bacteria include salmonella and E coli.
4. They follow the Chinese Government Herbal Pharmacopoeia guidelines of herb quality control for products, production methods, testing methods, fillers and strict standards of herb quality control. Their HPLC tests indicate that the herbs which they use have a very high content of active ingredients.
5. Lanzhou uses a three-step process to purify water used in all processes in the preparation of herbs. First the water passes through a sand filter, next through charcoal filters, and finally through an ionization process to remove heavy metals.
6. As a GMP factory, the air in manufacturing areas is filtered to remove dust particles and any other airborne contaminants.
7. All herbs are sorted and washed in a two-step tumbling warm water machine before production, using only purified water.
8. If herbs need to be dried after cleaning for further processing (slicing, pulverizing), they are dried at low temperature (below 80 degrees).
9. Production facilities follow traditional cooking methods and produce an extraction (tang or literally herbal soup) of about 80%. They use all stain-

less steel pressure cookers or ceramic-lined cookers. Some herbs are extracted individually because they may need special processing or have a different extraction time. Herb cookers hold approximately one metric ton of water and about 100 kgs of herbs.

10. The cooking process never exceeds 100 degrees Celsius, and water content is further reduced in a several step evaporation process to make a thick paste, which is done under 50 degrees Celsius in order to ensure that active ingredients are not harmed or damaged by excessive heat.

11. Volatile essential oils are captured in the cooking process and added back into the herb mixture after the liquid soup is strained to remove any larger particles.

12. The herb mixture is not freeze dried.

13. Pills are manufactured by chopping the dehydrated herb mixture into small pellets which are then placed into a drying pan where plant wax is added to create a smooth, easy-to-swallow pill. As of October 1996, Lanzhou produced 12 million pills per day.

14. All products are tested after completion of the manufacturing process and are tested by HPLC methods to ensure that the active ingredients remain and are still in the correct proportions. They test again for heavy metals, yeast and mold, and for pesticide residue.

15. Every batch of pills is also tested to ensure that they dissolve within the 45 minute requirement of the factory. 120 minute dissolution is required by the Chinese Government.

Lanzhou Foci factory has thoroughly tested their products and found that almost all have an active shelf life of eight years—but they use an expiration date of three years.

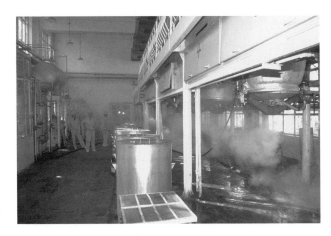

Herb cookers, Lanzhou

VISITING LANZHOU

In October 1996, I visited the Lanzhou Foci Herb Company for the first time. While there, I was given a complete tour of the company's facilities and was free to observe every step of the manufacturing process. I came away impressed by what I saw. Compared to factories and facilities in the U.S., the Lanzhou facilities are exceptional, surpassing every factory that I have seen to date in the U.S. in the production of herbal products.

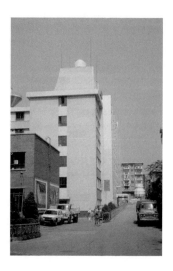

The people at the factory are knowledgeable and were helpful to me. I was impressed by their experience and the dedication with which they approach their work. They manufacture high-quality products and seem to be concerned that they continue to be on the cutting edge of technology so that they can continue their tradition of producing high-quality products.

Recently, they spent $3 million building a new factory in order to upgrade the quality and volume of their production. I toured this new facility prior to the grand opening and was favorably impressed with their efforts to remain a world class manufacturing facility. I have also seen independent lab tests of their products which support their reputation for good quality. I therefore feel confident in recommending the herb products manufactured by the Lanzhou Foci Herb factory.

They not only produce classic, time-tested herb formulas which have been shown to be effective and safe over the last several hundred years, but they follow traditional production values while using the most sophisticated manufacturing processes available. Additionally, they have nearly 70 years of experience producing these quality products.

Unfortunately, because of their reputation for high quality, Lanzhou products are widely counterfeited. When I go to herb stores, most of what I see are counterfeit products. The demand for Lanzhou products is very high because they are of such high quality—making them a likely target for counterfeiters.

HOW CAN YOU BE CERTAIN
THAT YOU ARE GETTING LEGITIMATE PRODUCT?

Lanzhou Foci products are exclusively distributed by just one company in the U.S.—Mayway Corporation of Oakland, California. Each legitimate product carries a Mayway code number on the top of the box. In October of 1996, I met with Lanzhou management and Mayway representatives at the Lanzhou factory, and we discussed changing the labels of Lanzhou products so that it would be more difficult for counterfeiters to copy. In October 1997, I observed the editing and changing of labels to make counterfeiting more difficult. These changes will probably occur after publication of this book and therefore cannot be included here. Look for notation of GMP certification on all Lanzhou labels in the future.

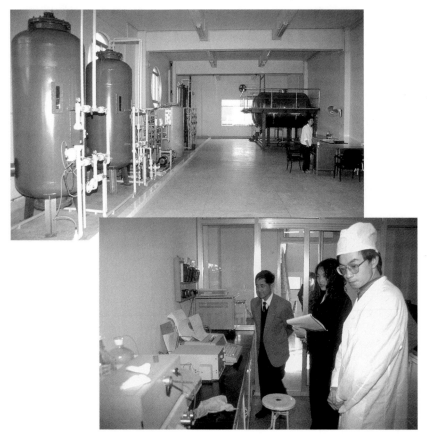

Top: *Water purification equipment, Lanzhou.* Bottom: *Quality control lab, Lanzhou*

49

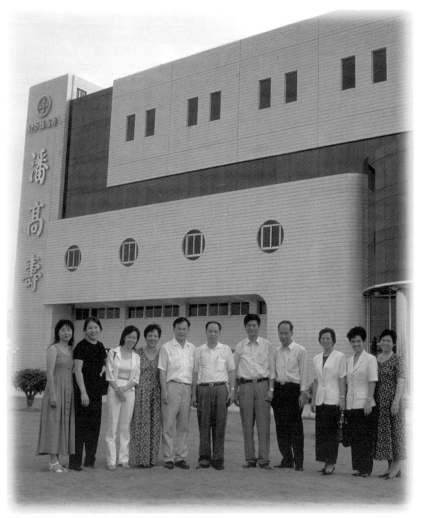

Guangzhou Pangaoshou Factory

4

WHAT IS GMP?

Good Manufacturing Practices (GMP) is a standard originally established for the U.S. manufacture of pharmaceutical drugs. This designation has since been adopted by herbal and pharmaceutical manufacturers in Europe and Asia. It is now being eagerly coveted by Chinese companies producing herbal medicines.

GMP standards establish certain basic guidelines which a factory must follow in order to be licensed to produce drugs or herbal medicines for specific markets. Requirements to qualify for GMP status vary from country to country, but it is generally recognized that the Australian Government's Therapeutic Goods Administration standards are equivalent to the highest International GMP standards in the world, higher than the American FDA. (See Appendix, p. 266, for copies of GMP certification.) As of 1997, the best factories in China have been scrambling to upgrade their facilities in order to be internationally certified GMP.

If a factory receives GMP certification, it can export its products to countries with demanding import regulations like Australia, Japan, Malaysia, and Singapore. As a consequence, international certification is very highly prized. At the time of this writing, it is estimated that no more than 10 factories in China have been approved for International GMP status. It is therefore a very exclusive designation.

In my visits to China in 1996 and 1997, I inspected a number of different facilities, some of which were GMP certified and some which were not. It was apparent to me that non-certified factories were inferior to certified GMP factories, which were cleaner, better maintained, and more organized. I have to say also that I was more impressed by the Chinese facilities than in my visits to American manufacturers.

What does this mean to the consumer? For those concerned with getting the best quality, International GMP certification is an objective assurance of the highest possible production values.

GMP standards include strict, technical protocols for manufacturing processes, sanitation, health and safety which must be rigorously followed. It also includes careful monitoring of production, detailed record keeping, and quality control standards which include inspection, testing, and recall procedures. These standards are exacting, time-consuming, and expensive, but they ensure the highest quality and highest production values.

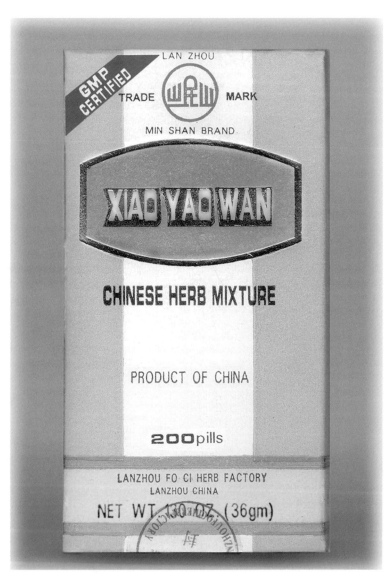

Photo of current package of Lanzhou Foci Xiao Yao Wan; look for packaging in the near future which will include GMP certified banner (see above) on upper left-hand corner of the box.

5

LANZHOU FOCI FACTORY PRODUCTS

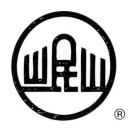

The following products are available in pill form from the Lanzhou Foci Herb Company under the Min Shan Brand. As mentioned earlier, Lanzhou Foci products are among the highest quality herbal products in the world and are therefore featured in this book. In the following section, I will discuss many of the formulas produced by the Lanzhou Foci factory.

Because the factory is GMP certified (see Appendix, p. 266) and because of its long history of producing high-quality products, Lanzhou Foci is unique in China. It has recently upgraded its production facilities and improved quality control to remain at the cutting edge of technological advancements in regard to herbal manufacture.

Of course, Lanzhou Foci is the most widely counterfeited of all the herb companies in China (see page 77). To ensure that you are getting the right products, see the opposite label of Xiao Yao Wan, as an example of correct packaging. Please note the logo on the box (also shown above on this page). Only purchase products which have this logo. Each legitimate product also has a Mayway code number on top of the box.

The factory is currently redesigning their labels to include recognition of GMP certification on the upper left corner of the box. This additional marking will appear at some time in the near future. Until then, the boxes will appear as it does on the left, without the GMP certified designation.

AN SHEN BU XIN DAN

Calm Spirit Nourish Heart Pills
The English-Chinese Encyclopedia of Practical
Traditional Chinese Medicine, Vol. #5
Chief Editor Xu Xiang-Cai, 1989 A.D.

Common Usage: Natural tranquilizer for anxiety, irritability, and insomnia.

Description: An Shen Bu Xin Dan is used to treat emotional troubles such as anxiety, irritability, emotional upsets, panic attacks, manic-depression (bi-polar disorders), uncontrolled emotions and resulting physical effects such as palpitations, insomnia, troubled sleep and dizziness.

Chinese Diagnosis: This formula works by helping to cool the blood and quiets the overactive, restless mind. It calms by nourishing the liver and kidneys which control the blood and fluids in the body. When the blood is cool and plentiful, the mind is calm because the heart and liver are properly nourished and cooled. Just as a radiator cools the engine in a car, the heart runs at the proper temperature when there is enough coolant. Without enough coolant, the car runs too hot, overheats and breaks down. This formula helps to cool internal heat which affects the heart which works with the liver to control the emotions.

Ingredients in the Formula:
Zhen Zhu Mu (margarita pearl) helps to pull heat down from the upper part of the body. A heavy mineral, Zhen Zhu sinks heat and supports the heart and liver.

Han Lian Cao (eclipta herb) supports the liver and kidneys, cooling heat.

Dan Shen (salvia root) cools the blood, calms the spirit, and supports the heart, eliminating irritability and restlessness. It also helps to encourage the flow of blood through the coronary arteries.

Tu Si Zi (cuscuta seed) strengthens the kidney Yin and Yang which supports all the internal organs and their normal function.

Ye Jiao Teng (polygonum multiflori vine) calms the spirit and nourishes the blood. When there is enough blood, all the organs are properly nourished and support the heart.

Shu Di Huang (prepared rehmannia root) tonifies blood to help calm the heart and mind.

Shi Chang Pu (acorus root) aids digestion and helps to calm the mind.

Wu Wei Zi (schisandra fruit) calms the heart and the mind.

Chuan Xiong (ligusticum root) improves blood circulation, particularly to the head where it can direct the calming energies of the various herbs of this formula.

He Huan Pi (albizzia bark) calms the spirit and is known as the "happy" herb.

Dosage: 8 pills three times per day.

BA ZHEN WAN
NU KE BA ZHEN WAN

Women's Department Eight Treasure Tea Pills
Women's Precious Pills
Women's Eight Treasure Tea Pills
Catalogued Essentials for Correcting the Body
(Zheng Ti Lei Yao)
Dr. Bi Li-Zhai, 1529 A.D.

Special Warning: This product is one of the most popular products in China and therefore counterfeits are very common. Counterfeits have many variant names including Ba Zhen Wan, Women's Precious Pills, Women's Eight Treasure Tea Pills. Before buying this product, make certain that it has Mayway code number printed on it.

Common Usage: Nourishes blood, improves digestion, regulates menstrual cycle.

Description: Ba Zhen Wan is the single most important formula for supporting and nourishing women who are blood deficient. It contains two smaller formulas, Si Jun Zi Tang (Four Gentlemen) to improve digestion and Si Wu Tang (Four Substances) to nourish blood and Qi.

It is especially important for women to promote the production of blood because they lose blood every month during menstruation. In the West, doctors often recommend iron supplements for anemic patients, but this is often inadequate because it focuses only on one nutrient. The richness of Ba Zhen Wan is that it helps to nourish all aspects of blood (red blood cells, white blood cells, platelets, plasma, fluid in the blood, etc.), and it regulates the movement or lack of movement in blood. It also aids digestion to improve the body's own ability to manufacture blood and assimilate the nutrients to build healthy blood.

If a woman loses a lot of blood during menstruation and has a busy schedule and perhaps eats a poor diet, then she could easily become undernourished. In fact, it is all too common for women to be anemic and blood deficient in this country without realizing it. A woman can also become very weak and deficient because of a chronic disease pattern or after delivering a baby.

Some of the symptoms of weakness and deficiency are a pallid or pale complexion, low appetite, shortness of breath, a very soft, weak voice, fatigue, light headedness, vertigo, anxiety, and possible heart palpitations.

Ingredients in the Formula:

Si Jun Zi Tang (Four Gentlemen) strengthens digestion. *Dang Shen* (codonopsis root), *Bai Zhu* (atractylodes rhizome), *Fu Ling* (poria cocos fungus), and *Gan Cao* (licorice root) improve digestive function, dry dampness and boost energy. Four Gentlemen also elevates the immune system. Blood is manufactured by the body from the nutrients provided by the food that we eat. When our digestion is good, the body produces healthy blood which nourishes all the cells in our system.

Si Wu Tang Wan (Four Substances) nourishes blood, helps regulate the menses, and prevents blood stagnation:

Dang Gui (angelica sinensis root) nourishes and regulates blood. It is important in assisting women both with hormones and with blood.

Shu Di Huang (prepared rehmannia root) nourishes blood to eliminate anemia. It also helps replenish yin body fluids which include hormones.

Bai Shao (white peony root) nourishes blood, stops pain, cramps and spasms. It helps to eliminate cramps by promoting the production of more blood and by helping the body to retain vital fluids which lubricate muscles, tendons and bones. Bai Shao is also an important herb to help normalize the liver function which controls blood flow during the menstrual cycle.

Chuan Xiong (ligusticum root) regulates blood, and helps stop pain, cramps and headache. It is a very important gynecological herb.

Dosage: 8 pills three times per day.

BAI HE GU JIN WAN

Lily Bulb Preserve Metal Pills
Lillium Tea Pills
Analytic Collection of Medical Formulas
(Yi Fang Ji Jie)
Dr. Wang Ang, 1682 A.D.

Common Usage: Stops cough, dry throat, coughing with blood.

Description: This formula is intended for chronic lung problems in which there has been a long-term cough, cough with blood or chronic dry, sore throat. It helps to moisten dry lungs and replenishes vital fluids in the lungs and throat.

In the Chinese five element system, metal is associated with the lungs, and this formula strengthens the function of the kidneys (water in the five element system) which prevents the depletion of metal (weakness of lungs; lung Yin deficiency).

Symptoms can include chronic cough, coughing with blood, wheezing, night sweats, a red, cracked tongue, hot palms and soles of the feet, dry and/or sore throat.

Chinese Diagnosis: This is called lung yin deficiency along with kidney yin deficiency. When the kidney yin is deficient, it can't steam water to cool the lungs and as a consequence the lungs become deficient and dry, causing a dry cough. This formula moistens the lungs and cools heat that causes coughing and sore throat.

This product can be used long-term to resolve the above conditions.

Ingredients in the Formula:

Shu Di Huang (cooked rehmannia root) and *Sheng Di Huang* (raw rehmannia root) both nourish yin fluids and blood, while Sheng Di Huang cools the blood.

Mai Men Dong (ophiopogonis tuber) clears heat from the chest and lungs and promotes the production of vital body fluids.

Bai He (lily bulb) nourishes the yin fluids of both the heart and the lungs, clears heat from the lungs and stops cough.

Chuan Bei Mu (fritillaria bulb) clears heat from the lungs and stops chronic coughing, strengthening the function of the lungs.

Bai Shao (white peony root) cools blood, nourishes blood and assures that fluids are retained when necessary by the body. It is astringent and is therefore able to contain the possible loss of essential fluids.

Dang Gui (angelica sinensis root) nourishes blood and stops cough.

Xuan Shen (scrophularia root) clears heat, cools blood and moistens dry, sore throat and dry mouth. It also provides moisture to the mouth and throat.

Jie Geng (platycodon root) normalizes the functioning of the lungs and improves digestion so that proper nourishment is able to reach the lungs and speed up the entire healing process. It also stops chronic cough and eliminates sore throat.

Gan Cao (licorice root) harmonizes the formula.

Dosage: 8 pills three times per day.

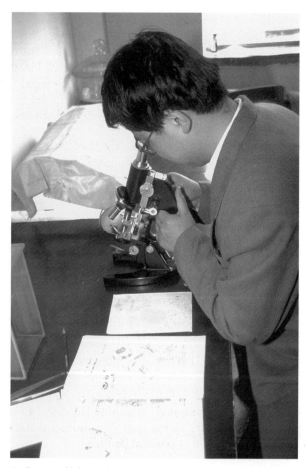

Quality control lab, Lanzhou

BAI ZI YANG XIN WAN

Biota Seed to Nourish the Heart Pills
Compilation of Materials of Benevolence for the Body
(Ti Ren Hui Bian)
Dr. Peng Yong-Guang, 1549 A.D.

Caution: Watch for counterfeits of this product.

Common Usage: Tranquilizer; calms restlessness, treats insomnia.

Description: This formula treats minor mental disturbances such as dream-troubled sleep, forgetfulness, mental confusion and anxiety.

Chinese Diagnosis: This formula helps to nourish the heart and therefore quiet the mind, which is controlled by the heart. Symptoms such as irritability, insomnia, difficulty sleeping and palpitations are often associated in Chinese Medicine with the heart not being properly nourished by the blood.

In this case, the kidney and heart are not working in concert. The kidney needs to properly steam fluids in order to cool the heat in the heart, and the heart needs to warm the kidney so that it can steam body fluids to prevent heat from becoming excessive.

Ingredients in the Formula:

Bai Zi Ren (biota seed) nourishes heart blood and helps to calm the spirit.

Gou Qi Zi (lycium fruit) nourishes the kidneys and nourishes the blood which will cool the heart.

Xuan Shen (scrophularia root) produces fluids which can cool the heart.

Mai Men Dong (ophiopogonis tuber) cools heat in the chest and calms the over-active, restless spirit.

Dang Gui (angelica sinensis root) nourishes blood. When there is sufficient blood, the organs are properly cooled and function effectively.

Shu Di Huang (prepared rehmannia root) nourishes the blood and yin fluids which calm the heart and the mind.

Fu Ling (poria cocos fungus) improves digestion and properly regulates the movement of fluids in the body.

Shi Chang Pu (acorus rhizome) opens the heart orifices to allow free movement of the blood and thereby helps calm the spirit.

Chai Hu (bupleurum root) sedates the liver, cools excess liver heat, and directs healing energy upwards to the heart.

Dosage: 8 pills three times per day.

BAO HE WAN

Preserve Harmony Pills
The Teachings of Zhu Dan-Xi
(Dan Xi Xin Fa)
Dr. Zhu Dan-Xi, 1481 A.D.

Caution: Watch for counterfeits of this product.

Common Usage: Indigestion, gas, bloating, motion sickness.

Description: This formula would be used when an individual overindulges in food or drink which causes an upset stomach. It can also be used when someone eats mildly contaminated food which causes simple diarrhea. It is especially good for children who experience upset stomachs or who do not seem to assimilate their food and remain skinny and underdeveloped.

Chinese Diagnosis: Bao He Wan is a basic formula for the treatment of food stagnation. Food stagnation appears in the form of a bloated, full stomach in which the food does not normally descend in the digestive tract and feels stuck, causing an uncomfortable feeling of fullness above the naval, unfortunately very common among young and old alike.

Symptoms include belching, heartburn, nausea, vomiting, little or no appetite, and possible diarrhea.

A variation of Er Chen Wan (see page 71), Bao He Wan can be used often and regularly. It is similar to Bao Ji Wan (Po Chai Pills) and Curing Pills, and is intended to be taken for simple indigestion caused by either overeating or from a weak digestive system that can't handle a normal meal. Some people have stronger digestive systems than others and therefore can eat larger, heavier meals. If the digestive system is not strong, even a small meal can cause an upset stomach. This is especially true as people age. The ability of the digestive system tends to weaken over the years, and older people often cannot eat large meals and must moderate their intake of food in order not to overwhelm their stomachs.

Ingredients in the Formula:

The formula, *Er Chen Tang* (see page 71), contains *Ban Xia* (prepared pinellia rhizome), *Fu Ling* (poria cocos fungus), and *Chen Pi* (aged citrus peel) and helps regulate digestion and to eliminate phlegm and dampness from the digestive system. Dampness and phlegm have sticky, stagnant qualities that impede digestion and slow the digestive process. One of the effects of Bao He Wan is to eliminate dampness and therefore speed up the digestion.

Shan Zha (hawthorn fruit) is especially effective in digesting meat and fatty foods. Modern research has shown that it helps lower blood cholesterol by breaking down fat in the blood stream.

Mai Ya (sprouted barley) helps digest grains like wheat which cause allergic reactions in some people and are difficult for the digestive system. The wheat protein, gluten, is particularly difficult for some to digest and is a common allergen in children.

Shen Qu (fermented leaven) is a fermented mix of herbs and grains which breaks down alcohol and several other foods that are heavy, sticky and seem to sit like a rock in the stomach.

Lai Fu Zi (radish seed) is effective in reducing sticky phlegm which is created by undigested starchy grains in the stomach.

Lian Qiao (forsythia fruit) works as an antibiotic on treat illness brought on by eating contaminated food or drinking unclean water.

Note: This formula can be taken often for chronic digestive difficulties, but any long-term digestive condition should be treated by a licensed practitioner.

Bao He Wan can also be used to treat stomach flu, but a better choice is Huo Xiang Zheng Qi Wan (see page 78).

Dosage: 8 pills three times per day.

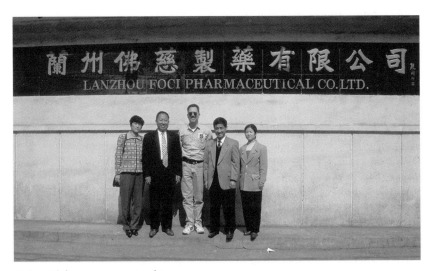

Author with factory managers, Lanzhou

BU ZHONG YI QI WAN

Central Qi Tea Pills
Discussion of Spleen and Stomach
(Pi Wei Lun)
Dr. Li Dong-Yuan, 1249 A.D.

Caution: Watch for counterfeits of this product.

Common Usage: Strengthens digestion, lifts prolapsed organs, stops chronic loose stools.

This formula is usually taken when someone is very weak, either following a prolonged illness or simply due to a weak constitution. It can manifest in three different ways:

Anemia in women with either spotting in between menses or recurrent menses (more than one period per cycle) with pale, thin blood.

Chronic diarrhea, or chronic loose stools with undigested food in the stools.

Prolapsed organs, such as prolapsed stomach, prolapsed rectum, prolapsed uterus, prolapsed bladder or hemorrhoids.

Other symptoms include chronic fatigue, fear of cold, pale face, pale skin, cold hands and feet, chronic nosebleeds and little or no energy for basic functions such as speaking or exercise.

Chinese Diagnosis: It is said that the Central (Zhong) Qi is weak and therefore cannot support the center of the body. This prescription is called Central Qi pills because central Qi controls the center of the body as though a tube extends from the neck to the bottom of the torso. Central Qi pills deal with conditions of weakness and deficiency in the middle of the body. When the central Qi is weak, the middle cannot be held up and this weakness can manifest in chronic diarrhea which is not caused by bacteria, but simply by the body's inability to digest food properly.

A variation of Si Jun Zi Tang (Four Gentlemen), Bu Zhong Yi Qi Wan is intended to aid digestion and to strengthen the middle Qi of the body.

In other chronic cases, some organs may prolapse, such as the stomach, uterus and the anus. The digestion may also be weak and unable to control the blood, manifesting in some bleeding disorders such as menstrual bleeding between menses or prolonged menses, nose bleeds and hemophilia.

Originally, this formula was used to cure those in the aftermath of a very serious disease when the body was exhausted and weak from severe illness. Over the years, its uses have expanded to treat certain forms of debility such as those leading to prolapsed organs, neurasthenia, anemia, muscle atrophy and digestive disorders.

Ingredients in the Formula:

Huang Qi (astragalus root), *Chai Hu* (buplerum root), and *Sheng Ma* (cimicifuga rhizome) lift the middle Qi of the body.

Dang Shen (codonopsis root), *Bai Zhu* (atractylodes rhizome), and *Gan Cao* (licorice root) are three of the four parts of *Si Jun Zi Tang* (Four Gentlemen) which help to strengthen digestion. (For a more complete discussion of the effects of Si Jun Zi, see page 178.) *Fu Ling* (poria cocos fungus), the fourth part of Si Jun Zi Tang (Four Gentlemen), has been removed because it has a downward draining function which works contrary to the basic intent of the formula which is to lift up energy.

Chen Pi (citrus peel) helps to regulate digestion and normalizes digestive function.

Dang Gui (angelica sinensis root) nourishes blood to promote overall well-being of the body. *Huang Qi* (astragalus root) and Dang Gui are a two-herb formula called *Dang Gui Bu Xue Tang* (Angelica Sinensis to Build the Blood Formula) which work together to build both blood and Qi which nourish all the organs of the body and helps to heal skin conditions as well as overall weakness.

Da Zao (black jujube date) harmonizes all the herbs and builds energy.

Sheng Jiang (fresh ginger root) aids digestion and warms the body.

Dosage: 8 pills three times per day.

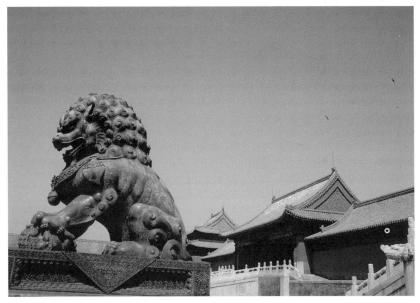

Forbidden City, Beijing

CHEN XIANG HUA QI WAN

Aquilaria to Disperse the Qi Pills
Modern Formula

Special Warning: Anyone feeling tightness in the chest or chest pains should see a licensed practitioner for proper diagnosis and treatment.

Caution: This formula may upset the bowels unless constipation is present.

Common Usage: Bad breath, constipation, abdominal fullness, belching, hiccup.

Description: This formula relieves congestion (stuck Qi) or pressure in the chest and abdomen. It improves digestion and bowel function, purging constipation and heat in the intestines.

Symptoms include a tight, constricted chest with pain and stuffiness, a feeling of fullness in the stomach. Also included are a pale face, fatigue, shortness of breath and poor digestion.

Ingredients in the Formula:

Chen Xiang (aquilaria wood) relieves chest constriction, releases stagnation and directs the energy downward away from the chest. It also helps to improve breathing by opening the chest to spread and diffuse stuck Qi. It also relieves hiccups, belching, and vomiting.

Dang Shen (codonopsis root) and *Bai Zhu* (atractylodes rhizome) strengthen the function of both the lungs and the digestive system so that energy can be improved. When digestion improves, energy perks up and the lungs grow stronger, so an individual breathes more easily and doesn't tire as readily.

Huang Qin (scutellaria root) clears heat from the chest and reduces inflammation, relieving a stifling sensation in the chest.

Da Huang (rhubarb root) directs the energy downward from the chest where it has become congested, purges the stool, and cools heat that may affect the chest.

Dosage: 8 pills three times per day.

CHUAN XIONG CHA TIAO WAN

Ligusticum to be Drunk with Green Tea Pills
Imperial Grace Formulary of the Tai Ping Era
(Tai Ping Hui Min He Ji Ju Fang)
Imperial Medical Department, 1078–1085 A.D.

Caution: Watch for counterfeits of this product.

Common Usage: Headache, common cold.

Description: This formula treats a headache which is contracted with a common cold. (For a more complete discussion of the common cold, see Ge Gen Wan, page 156 and Yin Chiao Jie Du Wan, page 121.) This formula is designed specifically to treat a headache that manifests on the back of the neck or on the top of the head, accompanying the symptoms of a common cold.

It can also treat some types of headaches that occur without a concurrent common cold. See below.

Chinese Diagnosis: A common cold attacks the individual from the outside. It invades the superficial layers of the body, the Yang meridians, predominantly on the head, the back of the neck and shoulders, causing stiffness and pain. In order to treat a common cold, herbs are taken to induce sweating. Sweating opens the pores, reduces the fever and encourages healing. Many of the herbs in this formula are diaphoretics and cause sweating.

Symptoms include fever and chills (with more chills and bodyache than fever), fatigue, slight dizziness and nasal congestion, usually with clear mucus. Some other types of headaches can also be treated, but caution is advised. [See note below.]

Ingredients in the Formula:
Green Tea: This formula should be taken with green tea because the properties of the tea balance and moderate the warm, drying herbs in the formula. Green Tea is cool and keeps the formula from being too warm. It also contains properties which stimulate the immune system and reduce inflammation.

Bo He (mint herb) clears heat from the face and eyes, alleviates headache and reduces fever. It is also a cool herb that balances the warm, dry properties of the other herbs in this formula. Bo He soothes the throat and stops cough. It also helps to calm irritability which is often associated with illness.

Chuan Xiong (ligusticum root) regulates circulation of blood, disperses wind and alleviates headaches on the side of the head and at the top of the head.

Qiang Huo (notopterygium rhizome) alleviates headaches, especially on the back of the head (the occiput), and relieves the pain of a tight neck, achy upper back and shoulders.

Bai Zhi (angelica dahurica root) helps eliminate headache on the forehead and above the eyes. It also dries nasal congestion, especially clear or white mucus

Xi Xin (asarium herb) stops headache pain above the eyes and on top of the head, as well as alleviates body aches. It dries nasal congestion and breaks up mucus stagnation in the nose to improve breathing.

Fang Feng (siler; ledebouriella root) treats headache, chills and achy limbs from common cold. In Chinese Medicine, it is said that wind carries the common cold and that there are several types of common cold, with wind-cold and wind-heat being the two predominant types. Fang Feng translates to mean "guard against wind," and it helps to protect the body from the "wind evil" which brings illness.

Jing Jie (schizonepeta herb) is antibacterial and antiviral and can be used for both major types of common cold, either wind-heat or wind-cold. Along with Fang Feng, it is often used to treat infections in the upper respiratory tract.

Gan Cao (licorice root) harmonizes the actions of all the herbs in the formula and directs the actions of the herbs into all the main meridians.

Note: This formula should not be used by a weak or anemic person with a dull headache that gets worse in the afternoon. Nor should it be used for headaches associated with anger, drinking, a red face or stress, or by people with flushed face or hot flashes. It is not a painkiller like aspirin or ibuprofen, so it will not be effective for acute conditions. It may take one to three days of regular usage to eliminate the headache and other symptoms associated with the headache. In order to alleviate future headaches, it should be taken for a longer period of time.

Dosage: 8 pills three times per day.

CONG RONG BU SHEN WAN

Cistanches Tonify Kidney Pills
Modern Formula

Common Usage: Lumbago, sore, weak lower back and knees, frequent urination, constipation from dry stools.

Description: This formula tonifies kidney Yang, the fire of life. If the body is a fireplace, wood is the vital substance or yin energy, while the flames themselves are the yang. Neither can exist without the other. As we age, the fire does not burn as brightly as it once did. This formula rekindles the fire of life.

It replenishes the vital Yin substances and Qi which are depleted over time.

Symptoms of Yang insufficiency include lumbago, impotence, sore, cold lower back and weak knees, constipation due to dryness, constipation of the aged, diminished vision, frequent urination, incontinence, dripping after urination, and excessive sweating.

Ingredients in the Formula:

Rou Cong Rong (cistanches herb) warms the yang fire of life.

Shu Di Huang (prepared rehmannia root) tonifies blood and vital yin fluids so that the fire doesn't get too hot. It supports the kidney Qi and balances the vital life force energy while helping to create Jing (vital life force essence).

Tu Si Zi (cuscuta seed) fortifies the kidneys, supports the yin and Jing and helps to retain the vital life force essence, which can leak out through excessive sexual activity or other dissipating behavior. Tu Si Zi relieves such problems as frequent urination, low back pain, ear ringing, impotence, and premature ejaculation. It also strengthens the liver and the digestive system, promoting both yin and yang energy.

Wu Wei Zi (schisandra fruit) supports the kidneys and retains the essence. It's most important function in this prescription is to contain the yang Qi which is provided by the other herbs. Wu Wei Zi retains the valuable nourishing qualities and supports the heart.

Dosage: 8 pills three times per day.

DA BU YIN WAN

Great Tonify Yin Pills
Teaching of Zhu Dan-Xi
(Dan Xi Xin Fa)
Dr. Zhu Zhen-Heng, 1481 A.D.

Common Usage: Nourishes liver and kidneys and clears heat.

Description: Like Liu Wei Di Huang Wan (see page 85), Da Bu Yin Wan treats Liver and Kidney yin deficiency, but this formula is much stronger in clearing heat. If Liver and Kidney yin deficiency are allowed to continue without proper treatment, the condition will manifest in very strong heat signs that can affect many areas of the body.

Unchecked Kidney Yin deficiency can lead to afternoon fevers, intense heat on the head such as hot flashes or flushed face, night sweats, irritability, heat and pain in the knees and legs.

Chinese Diagnosis: This is extreme Liver and Kidney yin deficiency. The yin fluids of the kidney are not sufficient to cool the heat of the liver and other organs of the body, permitting the heat to rise up to affect the lungs and the stomach. In order to reduce the heat, it is necessary to cool the internal organs with kidney water.

Ingredients in the Formula:

Shu Di Huang (prepared rehmannia root) nourishes the kidney and the liver, promoting the cooling properties of kidney water.

Gui Ban (fresh-water turtle shell) sinks the yang energy and cools the heat by nourishing water.

Zhi Mu (anemarrhena rhizome) clears heat and promotes yin fluids which cool internal body heat.

Huang Bai (phellodendron bark) clears heat from the lower part of the body, especially the kidneys.

Dosage: 8 pills three times per day.

DANG GUI SU WAN

Angelica Sinensis Pills
Modern Concentrated Single-Herb Formula

Common Usage: Regulates menstrual cycle, nourishes blood.

Description: Dang Gui nourishes and regulates blood and therefore assists women with their menstrual cycle. It is commonly used for women with pale complexions who have small, short menstrual periods (or no period at all) and women who are anemic.

Single herbs are not often used in Chinese Medicine, but Dang Gui Su is an exception because of the unique benefits of the single herb which is concentrated here to improve its healing qualities.

Note: It should not be taken during menstruation because it might cause excessive menstrual bleeding.

Dosage: 8 pills three times per day.

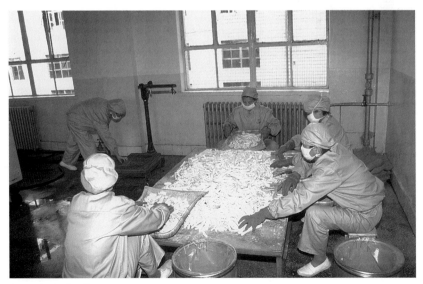

Sorting herbs, Lanzhou

DANG GUI WAN

Chinese Angelica Pills
Essentials from the Golden Cabinet
(Jin Gui Gao Lue)
Dr. Chang Chung-Ching, 142–220 A.D.

Caution: Watch for counterfeits of this formula.

Common Usage: Anemia, PMS, fatigue.

Description: Dang Gui Wan can be taken by women with anemia, temporary fatigue, irregular menstrual cycle, and PMS. Other signs and symptoms can include pale face, pale skin, difficulty gaining weight, inability to produce enough blood, and scanty, short menstrual periods.

Chinese Diagnosis: Dang Gui Wan nourishes blood, promotes more energy and improves digestion. By improving digestion, this formula helps to make more blood through better assimilation, making more nutrients available for the formation of blood. More blood means better energy and better functioning of the body.

Ingredients in the Formula:
Dang Gui (angelica sinensis root) nourishes and invigorates blood to prevent clotting and PMS. By promoting the manufacture of more blood, it creates more energy since the body is better nourished overall.

Chuan Xiong (ligusticum root) moves the blood and Qi and is very important for all gynecological problems. It also improves headaches associated with fatigue, late afternoon exhaustion, as well as the menstrual cycle.

Bai Zhu (atractylodes rhizome) improves digestion, dries dampness and improves assimilation of nutrients.

Da Zao (black jujube dates) tonifies Qi and harmonizes the formula.

Dosage: 8 pills three times per day.

ER CHEN WAN

Two Old Valuable Herbs Pills
Imperial Grace Formulary of the Tai Ping Era
(Tai Ping Hui Min He Ji Ju Fang)
Imperial Medicine Department, 1078–1085 A.D.

Caution: This product is very popular and widely counterfeited. I have seen many different versions and many different counterfeits.

Common Usage: Cough, clear or white phlegm in the lungs.

Description: Er Chen Tang is an important, classic formula in Chinese Herbal Medicine. Taken alone, the main use of this medicine is to remove excess phlegm and dampness from the lungs, to stop a cough and relieve a congested chest.

Major symptoms include thick and easily coughed up damp phlegm which is either white or clear. It can also be taken for bloating, nausea, vomiting, dizziness which is associated with poor digestion.

Er Chen Wan can also be used to treat difficult, chronic bronchitis with knotted phlegm that cannot be coughed up and which is usually stuck deep in the lungs. It can also be used for emphysema and any lung condition that produces difficult, sticky phlegm.

It is also the foundation for any formula which requires the removal of phlegm in order to facilitate healing. Depending on the herbs with which it is combined, it can be used to remove hot sticky yellow phlegm (Qing Qi Hua Tan Wan, see page 96), or it can remove dampness from the stomach and digestive system (Bao He Wan, see page 60).

Ingredients in the Formula:

Ban Xia (Pinellia rhizome) is the most important herb in the *Materia Medica* for the removal of phlegm. It also works to treat the source of phlegm. In Chinese Medicine, phlegm is often caused by a weakness of digestion which cannot properly regulate the fluids which are consumed. When dampness accumulates, it is stored in the lungs and begins to consolidate into phlegm. The longer that dampness remains in the body, the more sticky and hard to remove the phlegm becomes.

Chen Pi (aged citrus peel) helps to regulate the Qi of the stomach and all digestive energy. It gives appropriate direction to the flow of stomach Qi, stopping abdominal bloating, belching, nausea and vomiting. It assists in the stopping of coughs and in the elimination of phlegm.

Fu Ling (poria cocos fungus) is the most important herb in the Materia Medica for removing excess water and to channel the fluids into the right places of the body. It prevents the buildup of excess dampness and passes unwanted fluids out of the body.

Gan Cao (licorice root) harmonizes the functions of the digestive system. It also guides the actions of the herbs into the right meridians and it is used in many formulas in Chinese Medicine to harmonize and to improve flavor.

Sheng Jiang (fresh ginger rhizome) aids digestion and helps to break up phlegm stagnation in the lungs, bronchials, and nasal passages.

Dosage: 8 pills three times per day.

ER LONG ZUO CI WAN

Er Ming Zuo Ci Wan
Ear Ringing Left Kidney Support Pills
Tso Tzu Otic
Discussion of Widespread Warm Epidemics
(Guang Wen Yi Lun)
Dr. Dai Tian-Zhang, 1722 A.D.

Caution: This product is widely counterfeited.

Common Usage: Ear ringing (tinnitus), deafness.

Description: Ear ringing or tinnitus often occur without any apparent reason. It may sometimes be associated with having listened too long to loud music, or to a build up of certain types of fluids in the ear, but in reality Western doctors do not have a good explanation for its occurrence, nor do they have very effective treatment for this problem.

In Chinese Medicine, ear ringing and poor hearing are usually associated with deficient kidneys, especially in the elderly. When the kidney yin (essential body fluids) are insufficient, they cannot keep the active forces of energy (yang) under control. When there are insufficient fluids, the yang can rise up to the head where it causes complications, in this case ear ringing and deafness.

Ingredients in the Formula:

Ci Shi (Magnetite) and *Chai Hu* (bupleurum rhizome) help to control the hyperactive energy of the liver and to anchor liver Yang so that it doesn't rise up and disturb the hearing.

The foundation of this formula is *Liu Wei Di Huang Wan* (Six Flavor Rehmannia Tea Pills; see page 85) which treats Kidney yin deficiency. These six herbs nourish Yin fluids and strengthen the kidney function. In Chinese Medicine, the kidneys support the liver and the liver sedates Yang energy, preventing it from becoming hyperactive. When the liver is healthy, it anchors the Yang and normalizes it.

Shan Zhu Yu (cornus fruit) strengthens kidney function, helps to retain the vital life force essence (Jing), stops excessive urination and incontinence, preserving vital fluids.

Shan Yao (dioscorea root) improves digestion and appetite, assists weak lungs, and nourishes the kidneys.

Shu Di Huang (prepared rehmannia root) nourishes blood, yin and Jing. In nourishing blood, Shu Di Huang ensures that there is enough blood to nourish the skin, the hair and the nails as well as the ears. It also assists the heart and the liver which require an abundance of blood in order to function normally.

Fu Ling (poria cocos fungus) strengthens digestion and regulates vital fluids in the body, ensuring that they reach their proper destinations to lubricate and nourish.

Mu Dan Pi (moutan peony root bark) cools the blood and clears heat in the liver which burns up yin fluids. It also moves blood and breaks up heat-created blood stagnation.

Ze Xie (alisma rhizome) clears heat from the kidneys which burns up yin fluids and drains excess dampness that could contribute to stagnation.

Dosage: 8 pills three times per day.

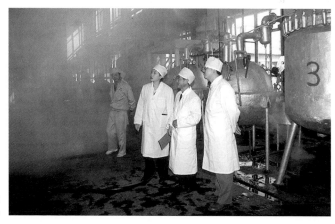

*Lanzhou
Foci Factory*

73

FU KE ZHONG ZI WAN
Women's Seed Planting Pills
The Book of Longevity
(Tong Shou Lu)
Author Unknown, Qing Dynasty, 1644–1911
[Based on: Jiao Ai Tang]
Donkey Gelatin and Mugwort Formula
Essentials from the Golden Cabinet
(Jin Gui Yao Liu)
Dr. Chang Chung-Ching, 142–220 A.D.

Special Warning: A woman who is pregnant should not take this formula without first consulting a licensed practitioner.

Common Usage: Stops bruising, stops spotting between periods, calms the restless fetus, promotes fertility.

Description: A variation of Jiao Ai Tang (Donkey Gelatin and Mugwort Combination), this formula contains herbs that nourish and regulate blood as well as strengthen the kidneys. The herbs in this formula help create a positive environment for fertility by warming the womb, promoting the production of blood, plus harmonizing and regulating female hormones. Like Yang Rong Wan, this formula also calms a restless fetus.

Ingredients in the Formula:
Si Wu Tang Wan (Four Substances) promotes the building and regulation of blood. See page 179.

Ai Ye (mugwort leaf) warms the womb, stops excess menstrual bleeding and cramps, and calms the restless fetus. It also combats threatened miscarriage and promotes fertility.

E Jiao (donkey skin gelatin) builds blood and helps to stop excess bleeding. It also nourishes the vital yin fluids.

Xiang Fu (cyperus rhizome) normalizes irregular menstrual cycles and controls the relationship between the liver and the digestive system, creating harmony in the middle of the body.

Du Zhong (eucommia bark) prevents miscarriage and strengthens the liver and kidneys, eliminating lower back pain, weak knees and frequent urination. It also helps to lower high blood pressure.

Xu Duan (dipsacus root) strengthens the liver and the kidneys which control the bones and muscles. Taking Xu Duan strengthens the lower back, bones and joints. It stops excessive uterine bleeding and calms a restless fetus, preventing bleeding during pregnancy and stopping miscarriage.

Huang Qin (scutellaria root) calms the fetus and clears excessive heat which may cause the fetus to become restless.

Dosage: 8 pills three times per day.

GU BEN WAN

Stabilize the Foundation Pills
Modern Formula

Common Usage: chronic dry cough, shortness of breath, dry mouth and throat, night sweats.

Description: Gu Ben Wan promotes original Qi, the source of all Qi in the body. Original Qi refers to the genetic essence which is the foundation of the life force. It is said in Chinese Medicine that the Yuan Qi, or source Qi, is our genetic bank account, the foundation on which our constitution stands. The kidneys are the repository of that vital life force energy.

This formula restores original Qi and Yin when are insufficient. We can deplete our Yin through various means, most commonly through self-destructive behavior such as doing drugs, eating improperly, or drinking too much alcohol. Other causes which exhaust Yin are over-work, especially mental strain, emotional excess and worry.

The herbs in this prescription also nourish Yin, the vital life force fluid which lubricates and cools excessive heat. The formula supports the lungs, stomach, and kidneys.

Ingredients in the Formula:
Tian Men Dong (asparagus tuber) supports the kidneys and the lungs, replenishing vital Yin fluids and reducing excessive heat. Signs of heat include dry mouth and throat, dry cough, flushed face and irritability.

Mai Men Dong (ophiopogonis tuber) supports the lungs and the stomach. When the stomach is strong and healthy, the body can rebuild and repair cells that break down. Healthy lungs are essential because they absorb oxygen without which we cannot function. When the lungs are healthy, the body also prospers.

Shu Di Huang (prepared rehmannia root) and *Sheng Di Huang* (raw rehmannia root) both nourish blood and yin. Shu Di more strongly nourishes blood while Sheng Di cools blood which is overheated. Heat in the blood can be seen in a rapid pulse rate. Both herbs fortify the kidneys which are the foundation of all life force energy.

Dang Shen (codonopsis root) strengthens the function of the lungs and digestion. When digestion is strong, vital nutrients are properly extracted from food and carried to the lungs which disperse them throughout the body along with oxygen.

Dosage: 6 pills three times per day.

GUI PI WAN

Kwei Be Wan
Angelica Longana Tea Pills
Wake the Spleen Pills
Great Spleen Restoration
Formulas to Aid the Living
(Ji Sheng Fan)
Dr. Yan Yong-He, 1253 A.D.

Caution: This product is widely counterfeited.

Common Usage: Stress, over-work, pensiveness, anxiety, anemia.

Description: This formula addresses the problem of over-work, over-thinking and over-studying. In fact, it is often prescribed to cure "student syndrome"—studying so much and so long that both the mind and body become exhausted. In Chinese Medical theory, when mental activities dominate a person, there are often digestive difficulties. Too much mental activity upsets the stomach and impairs digestion. As a consequence, the body does not derive the vital essence from food and the heart is not properly nourished.

In Chinese Medical theory the concept of the spleen refers to the entire digestive process, including the digestive functions of the liver, gallbladder, stomach, pancreas, spleen and duodenum. Since Chinese Medicine evolved before detailed anatomical studies of human bodies existed, doctors of ancient China did not have available to them some of the knowledge we have today. However, they were able to devise treatments that are still effective today.

Chinese Diagnosis: Gui Pi Wan treats heart and spleen Qi deficiency, with concurrent blood deficiency. If the digestion has been weakened, then the body will not produce enough good quality blood. Without enough blood, the internal organs are undernourished, in this case affecting the heart in particular.

Symptoms in men can include heart palpitations, insomnia, anxiety and fatigue. In women, symptoms may also include the above as well as easy bruising or menstrual disorders, such as spotting between menses or small periods.

A variation of Si Jun Zi Tang (Four Gentlemen, see page 178), this formula works to improve digestion while simultaneously calming the spirit, quieting the mind, elevating the Qi and nourishing the blood.

Ingredients in the Formula:

Si Jun Zi Tang Wan (Four Gentlemen): *Dang Shen* (codonopsis root) or *Ren Shen* (panax ginseng root), *Fu Ling* (poria cocos fungus), *Bai Zhu* (atractylodes rhizome), *Gan Cao* (licorice root) is the classic herb prescription for improving weak digestion.

Dang Gui (angelica sinensis root) and *Huang Qi* (astragalus root) combine to create a two-herb formula called *Dang Gui Bu Xue Tang* (Dang Gui Tonify Blood formula). They work together to nourish blood and elevate Qi, or energy (Qi is created from blood and then gives the blood vigor). By building Qi and blood, the body works better and more harmoniously.

Suan Zao Ren (zizyphus seed) and *Yuan Zhi* (polygala root) both help to calm the spirit and to relax the mind. Suan Zao Ren nourishes liver blood which helps to nourish the heart and relax the mind to encourage sleep. Yuan Zhi calms the restless mind and assists in normalizing heart function.

Long Yan Rou (longan fruit) nourishes blood and calms the mind, specifically by supporting the heart and spleen in times of over-work and pensiveness.

Mu Xiang (saussurea root) strengthens the spleen, especially at times when it is over-taxed by stress and too much thinking. It also improves digestion when strong nourishing herbs are being taken by someone with weak digestion.

Da Zao (black jujube dates) builds energy and harmonizes digestion.

Dosage: 8 pills three times per day.

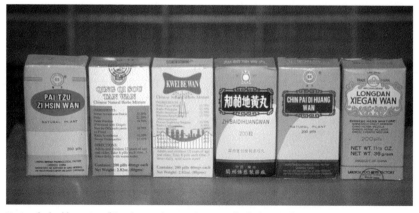

Various look-alike copies of Lanzhou packaging. Can you tell which one is legitimate?

HUO XIANG ZHENG QI WAN

Patchouli to Normalize the Good Qi Pills
Lophanthus Antifebrile
Imperial Grace Formulary of the Tai Ping Era
(Tai Ping Hui Min He Ji Ju Fang)
Imperial Medical Department, 1078–1085 A.D.

Caution: This product is widely counterfeited.

Common Usage: Summer cold, stomach flu, influenza

Description: This formula is commonly used for stomach flu or a summer cold with digestive difficulties. It can also be taken by those who are experiencing digestive difficulties associated with dampness: nausea, vomiting, fullness and sticky, loose stools.

A condition like this occurs most often in summer or in early autumn when an individual drinks lots of cold fluids when it is very hot. Digestion is impaired by excessive consumption of cold drinks, which weaken the immune system and create a condition of internal sluggish dampness in the intestines. The individual then becomes more vulnerable to catching a common cold or other sickness.

Huo Xiang Zheng Qi Wan fights stomach flu and includes herbs to eliminate digestive problems, phlegm and dampness.

Symptoms can include chills and fever, bloated chest, nausea, abdominal discomfort, loss of taste, little or no appetite, diarrhea, and/ or loose, sticky stools.

Ingredients in the Formula:

Huo Xiang (patchouli herb) is the chief herb in this formula and helps to transform dampness as well as release the exterior (expel the sickness evil), the two main functions of this formula. Dampness creates obstruction in the stomach and digestive organs which can cause vomiting or diarrhea.

Fu Ling (poria cocos fungus) and *Bai Zhu* (atractylodes rhizome) aid digestion by eliminating excess fluids and by drying dampness.

Zi Su Ye (perilla leaf) combats symptoms of the common cold such as chills, fever, headache, nasal congestion and cough. It also improves digestion by normalizing energy that may be stuck in the chest and abdomen which cause bloating and discomfort.

Bai Zhi (angelica dahurica root) reduces the pain of a headache, especially a headache located on the forehead, and dries dampness in the nasal passages.

Hou Po (magnolia bark) regulates the middle (stomach and digestive function), removes food stagnation, and discharges phlegm and dampness.

Da Fu Pi (areca; betel husk) eliminates stomach discomfort, reduces dampness and normalizes digestion.

Jie Geng (platycodon root) helps to normalize digestive function and to raise the vital essence, which is derived from food, to the lungs where it can be disseminated to the rest of the body. Jie Geng also strengthens the lungs and helps the lungs to spread defensive energy (Wei Qi) to the surface of the skin to drive away the external evil (pathogenic factor).

Chen Pi (aged citrus peel) regulates middle Qi (stomach, liver, gallbladder, pancreas, duodenum and spleen) and normalizes digestion.

Gan Cao (licorice root), *Sheng Jiang* (fresh ginger rhizome), and *Da Zao* (black jujube dates) harmonize digestion.

Dosage: 8 pills three times per day.

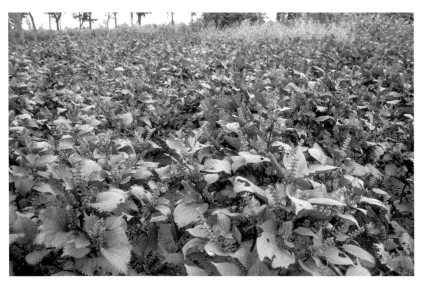

Zi Su Ye (perilla leaf)

JI SHENG JU HE WAN

Tangerine Seed Pills
Formulas to Aid the Living
(Ji Sheng Fang)
Dr. Yan Yong-He, 1253 A.D.

Common Usage: Hernia, testicular swelling.

Description: This is a condition in which the testicles enlarge and become painful. In some instances, the testicles will become very hard, sending pain up to the lower abdomen. If this condition persists without treatment, the testicles could become inflamed and irritated.

Chinese Diagnosis: The liver meridian wraps around the genital area. When cold and dampness block this channel, it creates stagnation of blood, Qi and phlegm, stunting the movement of fluids which congest in the testicles, causing swelling. If this condition persists, phlegm stagnation will turn into heat and become like an infection—red, swollen, hot and painful. It could eventually ulcerate and ooze a yellow fluid.

Ingredients in the Formula:

Ju He (tangerine seed) breaks up stagnation and masses, moves Qi and stops pain, especially in the hernia area.

Hai Zao (sargasso seaweed) and *Kun Bu* (kelp thallus) soften masses and break up stagnation.

Tao Ren (peach kernel) breaks up blood stagnation and masses.

Yan Hu Suo (corydalis rhizome) stops pain (especially in the lower abdomen), breaks up blood stagnation and moves Qi.

Chuan Lian Zi (melia fruit) breaks up stagnation in the liver channel and alleviates the pain from hernia.

Rou Gui (cinnamon bark) warms the meridians, warms the lower part of the body, especially the liver and kidney meridians which control the functions of the genitals.

Hou Po (magnolia bark) dries dampness, helps break up masses of dampness and phlegm, and directs the Qi downward.

Mu Tong (akebia stem) opens blood vessels in the lower part of the body, unblocking stagnation, reducing swelling and pain. It is a diuretic herb which provides an outlet for draining the dampness and phlegm which make up the swelling (mass).

Mu Xiang (saussurea root) moves Qi to break up phlegm stagnation.

Zhi Shi (immature aurantium fruit) breaks up masses, dissolves phlegm, and stops pain.

Yan Hu Suo (corydalis rhizome) stops pain in the lower abdomen.

Hai Dai (zostera marina herb) breaks up masses and lumps.

Dosage: 8 pills three times per day.

JIE GENG WAN

Platycodon Pills
Modern Single-Herb Formula

Common Usage: Chronic cough, smoker's cough, weak lungs.

Description: A single herb formula, Jie Geng Wan strengthens the lungs, aids digestion and helps stop coughs. It can also be taken for hoarseness or sore throat.

Jie Geng (platycodon root) is very mild and can be taken like food over a long period of time for any chronic weakness of the lungs, such as chronic cough with or without phlegm, for smokers with hacking morning cough, or minor coughing with blood.

Dosage: 8 pills three times per day.

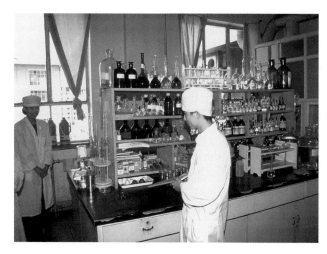

Quality control lab, Lanzhou

JIN GUI SHEN QI WAN

Golden Book Kidney Qi Pills
Golden Book Tea Pills
Essentials from the Golden Cabinet
(Jing Gui Yao Lue)
Dr. Chang Chung-Ching, 142–220 A.D.

Caution: This product is widely counterfeited.

Special Warning: This product should not be used by those with any internal heat signs such as red face or red eyes. Nor should it be consumed by those who anger easily or are irritable. Special care should be taken to make sure that this product is appropriate for the individual taking it. It is best to see a licensed practitioner in order to ensure proper treatment.

Common Usage: Impotence, infertility, prostate problems.

Description: People are born with different constitutions, some stronger than others, and some people simply do not inherit as much life force energy from their parents as others. Some people exhaust themselves through mental over-work, excessive physical and sexual activity and/or poor diet. Also, as people age, their vital life force energy naturally diminishes.

This formula replenishes the vital life force energy of the kidneys.

Chinese Medicine teaches that kidney energy is the foundation for good health. Kidney Qi is derived from kidney essence (Jing) and is replenished through maintenance of a healthy lifestyle and a healthy diet. For many different reasons, the life force energy is sometimes lacking and needs replenishing.

Symptoms of diminished kidney Qi appear as lower back pain, cold legs and cold lower back, tenderness of the lower abdomen, frequent urination especially at night, incontinence, impotence and infertility. Very common symptoms are lower back pain, weak knees and frequent urination. Awakening at night to use the toilet is a frequent problem with a large number of people as they age, especially for men after their forties. It is often associated with an enlarged prostate.

Jin Gui Shen Qi Wan replenishes both kidney yin and kidney yang as well as kidney Jing. All three are necessary in order to maintain a healthy body. Problems can occur when the three are weakened or imbalanced.

Chinese Diagnosis: Jin Gui Shen Qi Wan warms kidney yang, replenishes kidney yin and strengthens the functions of the kidney.

Ingredients in the Formula:

Fu Zi (aconite root) and *Rou Gui* (cinnamon bark) are hot herbs that feed the Life Gate Fire and restore kidney fire. Fu Zi improves the function of the heart, spleen and kidney yang, disperses cold in the deepest regions of the body and improves circulation. Rou Gui improves digestion, replaces lost vital life force energy, promotes circulation and improves stiff, achy joints.

The foundation of this formula is *Liu Wei Di Huang Wan* (Six Flavor Rehmannia Tea Pills; see page 85) which treats Kidney yin deficiency. The following six herbs nourish Yin fluids and strengthen the kidney function.

Shan Zhu Yu (cornus fruit) strengthens kidney function, stops excessive urination and preserves vital fluids.

Shan Yao (dioscorea root) improves digestion and appetite, assists weak lungs, and nourishes the kidneys.

Shu Di Huang (prepared rehmannia root) nourishes blood, yin and Jing. It also assists the heart and the liver which require an abundance of blood in order to function normally.

Fu Ling (poria cocos fungus) strengthens digestion and regulates vital fluids in the body.

Mu Dan Pi (moutan peony root bark) cools the blood and clears heat in the liver which burns up yin fluids.

Ze Xie (alisma rhizome) clears heat from the kidneys which burns up yin fluids and drains excess dampness.

Dosage: 8 pills three times per day.

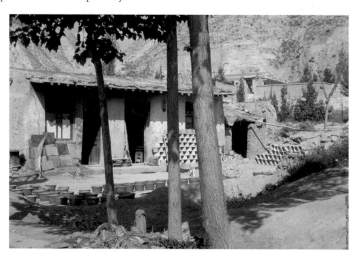

Pot factory outside Lanzhou

JIN SUO GU JING WAN

Golden Lock Pill to Retain the Essence Pills
Analytic Collection of Medical Formulas
(Yi Fang Ji Jie)
Dr. Wang Ang, 1682 A.D.

Common Usage: Impotence, premature ejaculation, male sexual dysfunction, frequent and/or excessive urination, bedwetting.

Description: This formula is intended to treat several problems related to male sexual function including impotence, premature ejaculation, wet dreams and other associated problems such as incontinence (the inability to control urine).

Chinese Diagnosis: The above symptoms are associated with an instability at the Gate of Life or a deficiency of kidney Yin and kidney Yang. When the kidney Qi (or kidney yang) is diminished, the sexual energy also declines.

Symptoms of weakened kidney function include lower back and knee pain, ear ringing, dizziness, blurry vision and incontinence. There is often a weakness of the kidneys and the liver together. In Chinese Medicine, the kidneys control the sexual energy, while the liver channel is directed around the genitals and therefore affects sexual function. This formula treats a basic weakness or deficiency of the kidney energy and the lack of control of the meng men (life gate).

This formula strengthens the kidney energy and helps the body to control the life gate, helping to retain the essence (Jing) which is found in the sperm and seminal fluid. By strengthening the kidneys, it helps the lower back and knees.

Ingredients in the Formula:

Lian Zi (lotus seed) and *Lian Xu* (lotus stamen) are astringent and assist the kidneys to contain essence. These herbs are common and easily found in the market place. Lian Zi is especially effective in calming the spirit and eliminating anxiety.

Sha Yuan Ji Li (astragalus seed) nourishes the kidneys and holds the essence. Its chief function is to stabilize the Gate of Life.

Qian Shi (euryale seeds) are commonly sold in Chinese markets and many dishes are prepared with them. They can be used as a food treatment to strengthen the digestion and the kidneys, also helping to hold the vital life force essence.

Long Chi (dragon teeth) and *Mu Li* (oyster shell) are both useful in calming the mind and storing the vital essence. They direct energy down into the kidneys and help to retain that energy so that it doesn't easily escape. They b gent qualities and contain calcium which helps to sede the restless spirit, relax muscles and aid peaceful sleep.

Dosage: 8 pills three times per day.

LIU WEI DI HUANG WAN

Six Flavor Rehmannia Pills
Six Flavor Tea Pills
Craft of Medicinal Treatment for Childhood Disease Patterns
(Xiao Er Yao Zheng Zhi Jue)
Dr. Qian Yi, 1119 A.D.

Caution: this is one of the most popular formulas in China. It is widely counterfeited. I have seen several different versions by different manufacturers.

Description: This formula has a wide ranging effect, addressing many different and varied conditions all arising from Kidney and Liver Yin deficiency. Six Flavor Rehmannia pills are the foundation for many other formulas. It is one of the most important enriching formulas in Chinese Medicine and can be taken long term for those experiencing the appropriate symptoms.

Liver and Kidney Yin deficiency is very common in modern society, and it is becoming more common. Such deficiencies are often created by a busy, overactive lifestyle, caused by excessive coffee drinking, excessive sexual activity, eating hot, spicy foods, not getting enough rest, excessive consumption of alcohol and drugs, cigarette smoking, and other speedy activities. In the body, there is a balance of yin (body fluids) and yang (the fire of life), and in our modern lifestyle there is always a tendency to do too much, to be too busy, to "burn yourself out." Living in excess burns up the yin fluids of the body which nourish the internal organs, tendons, and skin, hair and nails. Early symptoms of yin deficiency are dry scalp and dandruff, brittle finger nails, dry skin and a red tongue with little or no coating, often with associated cracks in the middle of the tongue body.

Symptoms of Liver and Kidney Yin deficiency are low back pain, weak low back and knees, pain in the heel or sole of the foot, excessive thirst, mental restlessness, headache, dizziness, blurry vision, night sweats, burning, frequent urination which occurs especially at night, and dark rings under the eyes.

One can have Liver and Kidney Yin deficiency without experiencing any of the above symptoms. A person could have some but not necessarily all of the symptoms and still have Yin deficiency. It is possible in the early stages to have only a few of these symptoms and for them to gradually become worse over time. Liver and Kidney Yin deficiency is a chronic condition, but it can occur in children manifesting in what is called "the five lates," slow development in standing, walking, speaking, and hair growth and in the appearance of teeth. It originally appeared as a pediatric formula to treat the five lates.

Ingredients in the Formula:

Shan Zhu Yu (cornus fruit) strengthens the kidneys, holds in the vital life force essence (Jing), stops excessive urination and incontinence. It also stops excessive sweating, either night sweats or sweating without exercise, and nourishes both the liver and kidney.

Shan Yao (dioscorea root) improves digestion, improves appetite, assists weak lungs, and helps to stop cough. It also nourishes the kidneys and helps strengthen digestion.

Shu Di Huang (prepared rehmannia root) nourishes blood, Yin and Jing. In nourishing blood, Shu Di Huang ensures that there is enough blood to nourish the skin, the hair and the nails. It also assists the heart and the liver which require an abundance of blood in order to function normally.

Fu Ling (poria cocos fungus) strengthens digestion and regulates the water passages in the body, ensuring that fluids reach their proper destinations and lubricate and nourish properly.

Mu Dan Pi (moutan peony root bark) clears heat, cools blood and cools heat in the liver which burns up yin fluids. It also moves blood and breaks up heat-created blood stagnation.

Ze Xie (alisma rhizome) clears heat from the kidneys which burns up yin fluids and drains excess dampness that could create stagnation.

Dosage: 8 pills three times per day.

LONG DAN XIE GAN WAN

Gentiana Clear the Liver Pills
Analytic Collection of Medicine Formulas
(Yi Fang Ji Jie)
Dr. Wang Ang, 1682 A.D.

Special Warning: This formula is often used to treat serious disease conditions, such as hepatitis, gall stones, and gall bladder disease. These conditions are best treated in a hospital or Chinese medical clinic. It is not recommended that anyone practice self medication in these situations.

Common Usage: Migraines, herpes, irritability, hepatitis, jaundice.

Description: This formula clears heat from the liver. It can also clear damp heat and liver fire. In this society in particular, liver heat is a very common problem. Liver heat is created by stress and intense constricting emotions which create obstruction in the liver. If such constriction is not relieved over time, heat is generated which, if allowed to grow out of control, can become liver fire.

Heat in the liver can either move down the liver meridian to cause problems in the genital area or it can move up to the head causing red eyes and headache. It can also remain in the liver area itself and affect the liver organ or the gallbladder.

The traditional uses of this formula were to treat serious diseases such as hepatitis, gallstones and gallbladder inflammation, but this formula can be used, however, by individuals to treat less severe symptoms such as irritability, red eyes, migraine headaches and herpes outbreaks.

Among the symptoms of liver heat are those that affect the head: Migraine headache (located on the side of the head, top of the head or behind the eye), ear ringing and deafness. Other symptoms can include those affecting the liver and gallbladder: Gallstones, inflamed gallbladder, jaundice and hepatitis. Symptoms affecting the genitals can include herpes, external genital discharge, vaginal discharge (foul smelling), urinary tract infection, kidney infection, testicle swelling or discomfort.

Diagnosing these difficulties can be very tricky, and it is better to rely on a practitioner in order to receive correct treatment. For example, a man with genital discharge might possibly have been infected by a sexual partner. On the other hand, he can have liver heat generated by stress which has moved down the liver meridian to the genitals to create damp-heat, causing the discharge. It is very important to make certain that he does not have a sexually transmitted disease.

Ingredients in the Formula:

Long Dan Cao (gentian root) is the chief herb in the formula. It clears liver heat, damp heat and liver fire (extreme liver heat). It can help red, painful eyes, red swollen sore throat, ear pain and swelling, and sudden deafness. It can also treat jaundice, genital discharge and pain, as well as vaginal discharge, especially if it is yellow and foul-smelling. It can relieve rib pain, chest and stomach pain from liver problems, as well as spasms.

Huang Qin (scutellaria root) clears heat and fire from the entire torso. It can treat jaundice, headache, red eyes and irritability.

Zhi Zi (gardenia fruit) clears heat, damp heat and liver fire. It is one of the main herbs for treating liver and gallbladder problems such as hepatitis, gallstones and gallbladder pain. It is also an important herb for relieving stress-related irritability.

Ze Xie (alisma rhizome), *Che Qian Zi* (plantain seed) and *Mu Tong* (akebia stem) all drain heat from the body through the urine. They are all diuretic herbs that clear heat from various parts of the body—Ze Xie from the kidney, Che Qian Zi from the liver, and Mu Tong from the heart.

Dang Gui (angelica sinensis root) nourishes blood which helps to cool the liver and to relieve liver Qi stagnation.

Chai Hu (bupleurum root) is one of the most important liver herbs; it works with the other herbs in this prescription to eliminate stagnation and cool liver heat.

Shu Di Huang (prepared rehmannia root) nourishes blood to enrich the liver.

Gan Cao (licorice root) harmonizes the formula.

Note: This formula should not be taken longer than a couple of months without the guidance of a practitioner because the herbs in it could cause some stomach discomfort. Hepatitis, gallstones and jaundice are very serious conditions. Proper treatment should be sought from a professional healthcare provider.

Dosage: 8 pills three times per day.

MA ZI REN WAN

Hemp Seed Pills
Discussion of Cold Induced Disorders
(Shang Han Lun)
Dr. Chang Chung-Ching, 142–220 A.D.

Special Warning: This formula should not be taken long term or during pregnancy because the herbs in this prescription drain energy downward.

Common Usage: Laxative.

Description: For those with dry stools, constipation, a bloated or painful abdomen, painful hemorrhoids from constipation. It can be taken for temporary relief of constipation from loss of body fluids, such as after childbirth or any type of heat condition which dries out the stool.

It can be distinguished from Run Chang Wan (see page 105) in that this formula includes herbs to stop abdominal pain.

Ingredients in the Formula:
Hu Ma Ren (flax seeds) replaces *Huo Ma Ren* (sterilized marijuana seeds) in this modern formula because of the drug stigma associated with marijuana. Hu Ma Ren is a natural laxative which provides oil to lubricate the intestines.

Da Huang (rhubarb rhizome) is one of the most effective herbal laxatives in Chinese Medicine.

Xing Ren (apricot seed) lubricates the intestines and directs Qi downward.

Bai Shao (white peony root) stops abdominal pain and spasms and, because of its astringent qualities, balances the formula so that not too much water is lost in the stool.

Zhi Shi (aurantium fruit) breaks up stagnation in the intestines and sends congested Qi downward, moving the bowels.

Hou Po (magnolia bark) normalizes digestion.

Dosage: 8 pills three times per day.

MAI WEI DI HUANG WAN

Ba Xian Chang Shou Wan
Eight Immortals Long Life Pills
Golden Mirror of the Medical Tradition
(Yi Zong Jin Jian)
Dr. Wu Qian, 1742 A.D.

Caution: This product is widely counterfeited.

Common Usage: Dry cough, chronic cough and bronchitis, weak lungs, dry skin.

Description: Another variation of Liu Wei Di Huang Wan, this formula helps to improve the functioning of the lungs, producing fluids for those with chronic dry cough, chronic bronchitis, excessive thirst, and dry skin problems. It is especially good for elderly patients who have become very deficient and have dry skin, dry cough, and other symptoms of aging.

Ingredients in the Formula:

Mai Men Dong (Ophiopogonis tuber) and *Wu Wei Zi* (schisandra fruit) help to nourish yin fluids in the kidneys and lungs. Mai Men Dong treats dry cough, assists the stomach and helps to relieve dry throat and dry mouth. It also moistens the stool and eliminates dry constipation. Wu Wei Zi strengthens the lungs and kidneys, stops chronic cough, and improves shortness of breath. Both herbs together work to calm the restless mind and eliminate irritability.

The foundation of this formula is *Liu Wei Di Huang Wan* (Six Flavor Rehmannia Tea Pills; see page 85) which treats Kidney yin deficiency. The following six herbs nourish Yin fluids and strengthen the kidney function.

Shan Zhu Yu (cornus fruit) strengthens kidney function, stops excessive urination and preserves vital fluids.

Shan Yao (dioscorea root) improves digestion and appetite, assists weak lungs, and nourishes the kidneys.

Shu Di Huang (prepared rehmannia root) nourishes blood, Yin and Jing. It also assists the heart and the liver which require an abundance of blood in order to function normally.

Fu Ling (poria cocos fungus) strengthens digestion and regulates vital fluids in the body.

Mu Dan Pi (moutan peony root bark) cools the blood and clears heat in the liver which burns up yin fluids.

Ze Xie (alisma rhizome) clears heat from the kidneys which burns up yin fluids and drains excess dampness.

Dosage: 8 pills three times per day.

MING MU DI HUANG WAN

Brighten Eyes Rehmannia Pills
Scrutiny of the Priceless Jade Case
(Shen Shi Yao Han)
Dr. Fu Ren-Yu, 1644 A.D.

Caution: This product is widely counterfeited.

Common Usage: Blurry vision, dry, shaking eyes, light sensitive eyes, night blindness.

Description: A formula for improving vision. The goal of the prescription is to support the kidneys. When the kidneys are strong, they properly nourish the liver which controls the eyes. Most often, vision problems are associated with liver imbalances, such as excess heat in the liver or insufficient yin fluids in the liver which allow the uncontrollable yang to rise and affect the eyes.

It can be used for chronic vision difficulties and should be taken long term in order to get the best results. It sometimes takes as long as a month to begin to see results when taking herbs, and a formula like this might have to be taken regularly for six months or more in order to achieve optimum results.

Ingredients in the Formula:

Ju Hua (Chrysanthemum flower), *Gou Qi Zi* (lycium fruit) and *Shi Jue Ming* (haliotis shell) have been added to the original formula. Ju Hua clears liver heat which affects the eyes, and Shi Jue Ming helps to anchor yang energy, which may be escaping the grasp of yin, allowing it to rise upwards to disturb the normal function of the eyes. Gou Qi Zi nourishes the blood to support the eyes and strengthens the function of the kidneys which assist the liver in improving vision.

The foundation of this formula is *Liu Wei Di Huang Wan* (Six Flavor Rehmannia Tea Pills; see page 85) which treats Kidney yin deficiency. The following six herbs nourish Yin fluids and strengthen the kidney function.

Shan Zhu Yu (cornus fruit) strengthens kidney function, stops excessive urination and preserves vital fluids.

Shan Yao (dioscorea root) improves digestion and appetite, assists weak lungs, and nourishes the kidneys.

Shu Di Huang (prepared rehmannia root) nourishes blood, Yin and Jing. It also assists the heart and the liver which require an abundance of blood in order to function normally.

Fu Ling (poria cocos fungus) strengthens digestion and regulates vital fluids in the body.

Mu Dan Pi (moutan peony root bark) cools the blood and clears heat in the liver which burns up yin fluids.

Ze Xie (alisma rhizome) clears heat from the kidneys which burns up yin fluids and drains excess dampness.

This formula treats excessive tearing, photophobia, red eyes and blurry vision.

Dosage: 8 pills three times per day.

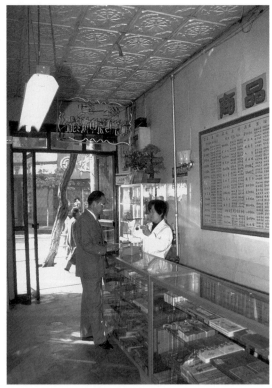

Herb shop, Lanzhou

MU XIANG SHUN QI WAN

Saussurea Root Normalize Qi Pills
Master Shen's Book for Revering Life
(Shen Shi Zun Sheng Shu)
Dr. Shen Jin-Ao, 1773 A.D.

Caution: This product is widely counterfeited.

Common Usage: Indigestion, stomach pain, constipation, irritable bowel syndrome.

Description: Digestive problems are a major complaint of patients worldwide. This formula addresses minor problems caused by improper eating habits, especially over-consumption of cold, damp foods which impede normal digestion. It also addresses common problems such as belching, heartburn and regurgitation of food.

It has a wide range of uses including normalizing digestion after the trauma of food poisoning or traveler's diarrhea. It can also assist in eliminating bad breath. It can be used for bloating, fullness in the stomach and a lack of appetite. It also helps to regulate and normalize bowel function.

It strengthens the stomach, soothes the liver and is used to treat chronic digestive problems like nausea and anorexia. It can also be used to treat early stage cirrhosis of the liver, irritable bowel syndrome and any number of digestive conditions which are untreatable by Western Medicine.

Ingredients in the Formula:

Mu Xiang (saussurea root) regulates and normalizes digestion. It creates harmony in the middle burner (stomach and digestive organs) and in the bowels. It stops bowel spasms and eliminates pain in the abdomen, chest and intestines.

Hou Po (magnolia bark), *Cang Zhu* (atractylodes lancea rhizome), and *Cao Dou Kou* (alpina katsumadai seed) dry dampness which makes intestinal function sluggish. While Hou Po normalizes the natural downward direction of digestive Qi, all three reduce bloating, nausea, vomiting, and loss of appetite.

Fu Ling (poria cocos fungus), *Ban Xia* (pinellia rhizome) and *Chen Pi* (aged citrus peel) make up three parts of the prescription, Er Chen Wan (see page 71), and improve digestive function. Together, they regulate digestion, drain excess and unnecessary dampness, clear phlegm and normalize intestinal function.

Qing Pi (green tangerine peel) breaks up stagnant energy and helps to regulate digestive function.

Yi Zhi Ren (alpinia seed), *Wu Zhu Yu* (evodia fruit) and *Gan Jiang* (dried ginger rhizome) all warm the stomach and digestion. Icy drinks and cold food, such as ice cream, damage the digestion and keep the body from properly assimilating food. These three herbs warm the digestion and restore the digestive fire that breaks down the food in the body so that it can be properly transformed into energy and vital nutrients.

Dang Gui (angelica sinensis root) warms and moves the blood to improve circulation and help digestion. In the digestive process, when food enters the stomach and intestines, the body diverts blood and Qi to the digestive organs in order to extract as much of the beneficial nutrients as possible. Improving blood circulation therefore improves digestion.

Zhi Shi (aurantium fruit) breaks up stagnation in the digestive system and encourages normal flow of digestive energy downward.

Ze Xie (alisma rhizome) promotes the movement of water in the body and drains dampness through urination. It also clears heat from the lower burner (urinary bladder, kidney, small intestine, large intestine).

Sheng Ma (cimicifuga rhizome) and *Chai Hu* (bupleurum root) assist in moving Qi upwards into the lungs where it can be properly dispersed throughout the body. Chai Hu protects the liver and regulates the liver Qi which often becomes stagnant and interferes with normal digestion.

This prescription has herbs that direct energy both up and down in the digestive system so that no stagnation can occur in the intestines. There are herbs to lift energy when the downward movement is excessive, as in diarrhea, and herbs which direct energy downward when energy and feces are stagnant above.

Dosage: 8 pills three times per day.

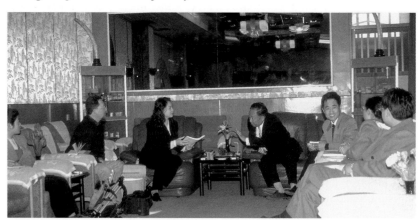

The author meeting with factory managers, Lanzhou

QI JU DI HUANG WAN

Lycium and Chrysanthemum Tea Pills
Precious Mirror for the Advancement of Medicine
(Yi Ji Bao Jian)
Dr. Dong Xi-Yuan, 1777 A.D.

Caution: This product is widely counterfeited.

Common Usage: Blurry vision, night blindness, red, dry eyes.

Description: This formula improves vision, supports the liver which controls the eyes, and nourishes the kidneys.

Ingredients in the Formula:

Gou Qi Zi (lycium fruit) and *Ju Hua* (chrysanthemum flower) support and heal the eyes. Gou Qi Zi is an important herb for nourishing the eyes and for building blood. It assists the liver which stores the blood and controls the eyes. Ju Hua clears heat from the liver and cools the blood; Ju Hua has actions that direct healing energy upwards to the eyes.

The foundation of this formula is *Liu Wei Di Huang Wan* (Six Flavor Rehmannia Tea Pills; see page 85) which treats Kidney yin deficiency. The following six herbs nourish Yin fluids and strengthen the kidney function.

Shan Zhu Yu (cornus fruit) strengthens kidney function, stops excessive urination and preserves vital fluids.

Shan Yao (dioscorea root) improves digestion and appetite, assists weak lungs, and nourishes the kidneys.

Shu Di Huang (prepared rehmannia root) nourishes blood, Yin and Jing. It also assists the heart and the liver which require an abundance of blood in order to function normally.

Fu Ling (poria cocos fungus) strengthens digestion and regulates vital fluids in the body.

Mu Dan Pi (moutan peony root bark) cools the blood and clears heat in the liver which burns up yin fluids.

Ze Xie (alisma rhizome) clears heat from the kidneys which burns up yin fluids and drains excess dampness.

This formula can be used long term for anyone with chronic visual difficulties except conjunctivitis, which manifests with red, swollen eyes. Use Ming Mu Shang Qing Pian for conjunctivitis (See page 240).

Dosage: 8 pills three times per day.

QING QI HUA TAN WAN

Pinellia Expectorant Pills
Clear Qi and Transform Phlegm Pill
Clean Air Tea Pills
Investigation of Medical Formulas
(Yi Fang Kao)
Dr. Wu Kun, 1584 A.D.

Caution: This is a very popular product in China and is commonly available only in counterfeit form. Make sure this product has a Mayway code number on the top of the box.

Special Warning: In serious disease conditions such as asthma and pneumonia, consult a licensed practitioner.

Common Usage: Bronchitis.

Description: This prescription is very popular and commonly used because it treats hot phlegm stagnation in the lungs—bronchitis, both acute and chronic. It may also be used to treat pneumonia and asthma with hot, yellow, sticky phlegm that is difficult to cough up and clear out of the lungs.

This formula clears heat from the lungs and helps to remove phlegm which is knotted or stuck in the lungs causing coughing and wheezing, pain in the chest with possible bloating, or fullness in the chest.

Ingredients in the Formula:

Jiang Ban Xia (prepared pinellia rhizome), *Chen Pi* (aged citrus peel) and *Fu Ling* (poria cocos fungus) comprise three parts of *Er Chen Wan* (see page 71). It clears phlegm and dampness from the lungs and helps to normalize the proper direction of lung Qi. It will also normalize digestion to remove phlegm from the body and therefore reduce phlegm congestion in the lungs.

The addition of *Dan Nan Xing* (prepared arisaema rhizome) and *Zhi Shi* (immature aurantium fruit) changes the formula to *Dao Tan Tang* (Guide Out Phlegm Decoction) which is stronger in breaking up knotted phlegm stagnation which is sticky, yellow and difficult to cough up. Dan Nan Xing dries phlegm and dampness and relieves bloating and discomfort of the chest. Zhi Shi breaks up stagnation with phlegm and gas, directs Qi downward and stops spasms.

Huang Qin (scutellaria root) and *Shuang Gua Lou Ren* (trichosanthis seed frost) both clear heat from the lungs and help to dissolve sticky phlegm. Huang Qin fights bacterial infection, killing toxins, and Gua Lou Ren purges thick, knotted phlegm. Both herbs can be used to treat lung abscess and a painful, bloated chest.

Xing Ren (apricot kernel) stops asthma, normalizes the proper direction of lung energy and moves the stool. When there is heat and phlegm stagnation in the lungs, there is also often an accompanying constipation which can be more easily eliminated after the lubrication of Xing Ren. When the bowels move freely, it helps to loosen up stagnation in the lungs.

Sheng Jiang (fresh ginger rhizome) improves digestion and dissolves phlegm stagnation in the lungs, bronchials, and nasal passages.

Dosage: 6 pills three times per day.

REN SHEN JIAN PI WAN

Ginseng Tonify the Spleen Pills
Standards of Patterns and Treatment
(Zheng Shi Shun Sheng)
Dr. Wang Ken-Tang, 1602 A.D.

Caution: This product is available in counterfeit form.

Common Usage: Anorexia, weak digestion.

Description: Ren Shen Jian Pi Wan strengthens the digestive system. It is intended for individuals who have very weak digestion and are not able to digest food well, thus creating a problem in which food stagnates in the stomach and intestines. It can be used in any condition of impaired digestion.

The symptoms of this problem are loss of weight, poor appetite and bloating. When an individual has poor digestion, they often are unable to digest food effectively, so a meal may just sit in the stomach. The individual has little appetite due to a sensation of fullness caused by undigested food that is stuck in the digestive system. Since food is not being digested or assimilated, there is weight loss. This situation can be accompanied by indigestion, loose stools, diarrhea, sometimes with undigested food particles, and/or constipation.

This formula can be used for a number of digestive diseases, such as psychosomatic eating disorders, anorexia, gastritis, intestinal prolapse, colitis and irritable bowel syndrome.

Ingredients in the Formula:
Dang Shen (codonopsis root) nourishes digestive energy as well as the overall Qi of the body. *Ren Shen* (panax ginseng root) is the strongest of all the herbs for elevating the Qi of the body, strengthening both the lungs and digestive organs. Dang Shen also strengthens the lungs and digestion, but it isn't as strong or as expensive as Ren Shen and is substituted for Ren Shen here because it is less expensive.

Bai Zhu (atractylodes rhizome) strengthens the digestive system and dries dampness which accumulates when the digestive system is not functioning well.

Shan Zha (hawthorn fruit) helps to digest meat and fatty foods which are especially hard on the stomach. When heavy, greasy, oily foods are eaten and the digestive system is weak, food sits heavily in the stomach and is difficult to move.

Mai Ya (sprouted barley) helps to digest grains such as wheat, barley and rye. Wheat especially is difficult for many people to digest and this formula is recommended to those who have food allergies. Allergic reactions to certain foods may well be more a problem of digestion and assimilation than an actual allergy to a particular food.

Chen Pi (aged citrus peel) helps to regulate digestion, by moving Qi downward in its normal direction.

Zhi Shi (aurantium fruit) breaks up stagnation and moves energy downward into the intestines, harmonizing the digestive tract.

Dosage: 6 pills three times per day.

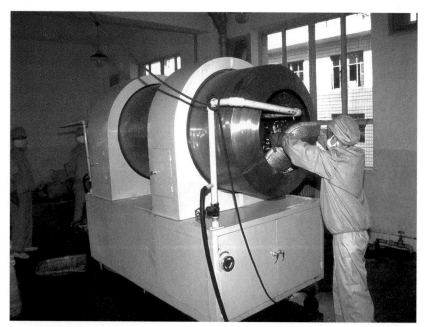

Herb sterilization equipment, Lanzhou

SHEN QI DA BU WAN

Codonopsis and Astragalus Lift the Qi Pills
Modern Formula

Caution: This product is widely counterfeited.

Common Usage: Fatigue, lack of energy, low immune system.

Description: *Dang Shen* (codonopsis root) improves digestion and strengthens lung function so that the body can better utilize oxygen. By improving digestion, the body generates adequate blood which in turn nourishes all the organs and the skin, carrying nutrients and vital fluids to every cell in the body. In assisting the digestive system and the lungs, Dang Shen promotes normal body function and builds Qi.

Huang Qi (astragalus root) strengthens digestion, builds the immune system and helps to produce blood. For those who experience recurrent common colds, Huang Qi helps to protect against infections. It is also beneficial for the treatment of general fatigue.

Ingredients in the Formula:
Huang Qi (astragalus root) and *Dang Shen* (codonopsis root).

Modern Research on the Immune System
Both of these herbs have been widely studied in modern China, and recent research has shown them to be very effective in boosting both cellular and humoral immunity. Dang Shen increases the T cell levels of the blood while Huang Qi increases macrophages (cells that ingest bacteria), increasing the body's ability to neutralize foreign invaders. They both promote the production of B cells and anti-bodies.

Huang Qi stimulates the production of interferon and fights viral infections. It promotes the production of lymphocytes and increases the production of all types of white blood cells. It has been used to treat influenza and infections in the mucus membranes of the nose and lungs for more than two thousand years.

See Yu Ping Feng San (Jade Screen Pills, page 201) for a prescription to build the immune system and prevent recurrent common cold.

Dosage: 8 pills three times per day.

SHEN QI WU WEI ZI WAN

Codonopsis, Astragalus, and Schisandra Pills
Modern Formula

Common Usage: Improves energy, boosts immunity, stops excessive sweating.

Description: This formula lifts energy, reduces excessive sweating—night sweats, spontaneous sweating, sweating easily from exertions—while calming nervousness and strengthening the immune system.

Note: Energy "boosters" have been very popular the past few years. These products usually contain herbs such as *Ma Huang* (ephedra), *guarana* (which contains caffeine) and *Ren Shen* (panax ginseng root). Stimulants are commonly abused in our contemporary world and are not beneficial to health when taken in excess or without supporting herbs to balance the excessive stimulating properties.

This formula is a balanced, gentle medicine which elevates energy, calms the nervous mind, and stimulates the immune system.

Ingredients in the Formula:

Dang Shen (codonopsis root) and *Huang Qi* (astragalus root) tonify the body's Qi, improving energy and athletic performance. Both herbs are well known for their ability to fortify immunity (see Shen Qi Da Bu Wan, page 99). These herbs are renowned in China for their effectiveness in improving overall energy and strengthening the function of lungs to boost endurance as well as improve digestion, increase assimilation of nutrients and utilize the energy in food.

Wu Wei Zi (schisandra fruit) calms the restless spirit, stops sweating to preserve the vital life force essence, and supports the kidneys, which provide the foundation for all bodily functions.

Suan Zao Ren (zizyphus fruit) promotes the production of liver blood which supports both the heart and the liver. In the five-element Chinese theory, wood nourishes fire, so liver blood (wood) promotes the heart (fire) by providing the heart with sufficient blood to nourish the heart muscle, supply the heart with oxygen, and cool the over-stimulated heart and mind. When there is insufficient blood, the heart has to work excessively which makes it overactive and therefore overheated. Along with Wu Wei Zi, Suan Zao Ren protects the heart and calms the mind to improve sleep, eliminate insomnia and irritability.

Dosage: 8 pills three times per day.

SHI CHUAN DA BU WAN

Ten Herb Great Nourishing Pills
Shi Quan Da Bu Wan
Shih Chuan Ta Pu Wan
Ten Flavor Tea Pills
Imperial Grace Formulary of the Tai Ping Era
(Tai Ping Hui Min He Ji Ju Fang)
Imperial Medical Department, 1078–1085 A.D.

Warning: This formula should not be taken by anyone who has heat signs, such as hot flashes, low grade fever, hot palms and soles of the feet or flushed face.

Caution: This product is widely counterfeited.

Common Usage: Fatigue, chronic illness, weakness, recovery from childbirth.

Description: This is a variation of Ba Zhen Wan (Eight Treasure Tea Pills; see page 55) with the addition of *Rou Gui* (cinnamon bark) and *Huang Qi* (astragalus root). It has the same actions as Ba Zhen Wan, nourishing and regulating blood, plus the warming and the stronger fortifying actions of the additional herbs. It may be used long term for those who are weak and anemic or those who have cold hands and feet. Other symptoms may include chronic coughing, reduced appetite and weakness of the lower back, legs, knees and ankles.

Ingredients in the Formula:
Rou Gui (cinnamon bark) warms the kidneys and fortifies kidney yang, strengthening the life force energy which promotes the nourishment of both Qi and blood.

Huang Qi (astragalus root) improves digestion, lifts energy and spirit, protects against the common cold and heals the body after loss of blood, especially after childbirth.

Dang Shen (codonopsis root), *Bai Zhu* (atractylodes rhizome), *Fu Ling* (poria cocos fungus), and *Gan Cao* (licorice root) improve digestive function, dry dampness and boost energy. These four herbs also improve the immune system. Blood is manufactured by the body from the nutrients provided by the food that we eat. When our digestion is good, the body produces healthy blood which nourishes all the cells in our system.

Dang Gui (angelica sinensis root) nourishes and regulates blood. It is important in assisting women both with hormones and with blood.

Shu Di Huang (prepared rehmannia root) nourishes blood to eliminate anemia. It also helps replenish yin body fluids which include hormones.

Bai Shao (white peony root) nourishes blood, stops pain, cramps and spasms. It helps to eliminate cramps by promoting the production of more blood and by helping the body to retain vital fluids which lubricate muscles, tendons and bones. Bai Shao is also an important herb to help normalize the liver function which controls blood flow during the menstrual cycle.

Chuan Xiong (ligusticum root) regulates blood, and helps stop pain, cramps and headache. It is a very important gynecological herb.

Dosage: 8 pills three times per day.

SHU GAN WAN

Smooth Liver Pills
Dr. Zhu Tian-Bi
Ming Dynasty, 1368–1644 A.D.
[Based on: Si Ni San]
Frigid Extremities Powder
Discussion of Cold Induced Disorders
(Shang Han Lun)
Dr. Chang Chung-Ching, 142–220 A.D.

Caution: This is widely counterfeited.

Common Usage: Reduces stress, aids digestion, normalizes menses, reduces PMS.

Description: Shu Gan Wan is designed to alleviate emotional congestion which traps the warmth of the body internally and will not allow it to flow to the hands and feet. Shu Gan Wan can be taken by anyone with emotional stress which is affecting digestion, causing alternating diarrhea and constipation, bloating, chest pain or pain in the liver and gallbladder area.

Chinese Diagnosis: The conditions mentioned above are the result of liver attacking the spleen, a very common diagnosis in Chinese Medical clinics here in the U.S. and in China. When one experiences a great deal of stress, the free flow of Qi in the liver is restricted. Under stress, people are said to become "uptight," or tense. When there is internal tension, Qi is bound up and doesn't flow freely or harmoniously. It can invade the chest, stomach or abdomen where it normally wouldn't go, interfering with digestion and causing pain.

Symptoms of liver Qi stagnation can be discomfort of the chest, belching, bloating, indigestion, alternating loose stools and constipation, menstrual cramps and PMS. Stress, PMS and digestive problems are common in our society and often are the direct result of Liver Qi stagnation.

This formula calms and sedates the liver which is said to "attack" the stomach and to cause stagnation in the digestive tract, creating bloating, fullness, belching, and sometimes vomiting. When stagnation occurs, proper digestion is inhibited causing pain and discomfort.

Shu Gan Wan also is a very important formula for regulating the menses. The liver controls menstrual blood, and anything that constricts the normal function of liver blood will impair the menses. This is especially true of emotional conditions such as depression, anxiety and irritability. Coffee congests the liver and blocks the free flow of blood and Qi, which causes menstrual difficulties.

Ingredients in the Formula:
Shu Gan Wan is an adaptation of the famous prescription, *Si Ni San* (Frigid Extremities Powder) and contains *Chai Hu* (bupleurum root), *Bai Shao* (white peony root), *Zhi Ke* (aurantium fruit), and *Gan Cao* (licorice root). Si Ni San encourages normal circulation of the liver Qi, regulates the menstrual cycle and warms the hands and feet. It releases internal heat which is trapped inside the body and encourages the free flow of warming Yang Qi to the hands and feet.

Qing Pi (tangerine peel), *Xiang Yuan* (citrus xiang yuan) and *Chen Pi* (aged citrus peel) regulate the energy of digestion, help to dry dampness, relieve stress and reduce stagnation in the digestive tract. Chen Pi directs the energy of digestion downward and assists both the lungs and the spleen. It is an especially important herb in prescriptions because it prevents other herbs from stagnating in the stomach and intestines. Qing Pi is more effective in breaking up liver Qi stagnation (emotional constriction) and in stopping pain.

Xiang Fu (cyperus rhizome), *Chen Xiang* (aquilaria wood) and *Tan Xiang* (sandalwood) all help to regulate the free flow of energy in the chest and stomach. Xiang Fu creates harmony between the liver and the spleen and normalizes the menses. Chen Xiang moves energy downward and stops pain in the chest and abdomen. Tan Xiang regulates energy in the chest and abdomen.

Yan Hu Suo (corydalis rhizome) stops pain in the chest, abdomen and lower torso. Yan Hu Suo reduces menstrual cramps and any pain in the upper or lower abdomen.

Mu Dan Pi (moutan peony root bark) clears heat from the blood and helps to break up blood stagnation. It is especially useful for women with clots and pain before menstruation, especially if they show signs of heat. These signs include hot flashes, night sweats, red cheeks, heavy menstrual flow with bright red blood, and a short cycle under 28 days. It clears heat from the liver and is useful when headaches accompany the menses.

Bai Dou Kou (white cardamon fruit) and *Sha Ren* (amomum fruit) aid digestion by eliminating stagnant dampness that may block normal digestive function. They both direct the normal flow of Qi in the digestive tract and warm the digestive fire.

Hou Po (magnolia bark) directs the energy of digestion downward, stopping vomiting, belching and hiccups. These symptoms occur when the normal downward flow of Qi is constricted either by dampness or by the invasion of the stomach by the liver. This invasion is like an emotional blockage and backs up normal Qi forcing it to go upwards, creating a situation where the Qi is rebellious, moving in the opposite direction from normal.

Mu Xiang (saussurea root) harmonizes digestion, improves intestinal function, and reduces abdominal pain, especially pain that is associated with stagnant bowels.

Fo Shou (finger citron fruit) regulates the liver and benefits digestion, reducing abdominal pain, chest pain, and bloating.

Jiang Huang (tumeric rhizome) regulates the blood, reduces pain and inflammation, and relaxes the shoulders where tension is often stored.

Dosage: 8 pills three times per day.

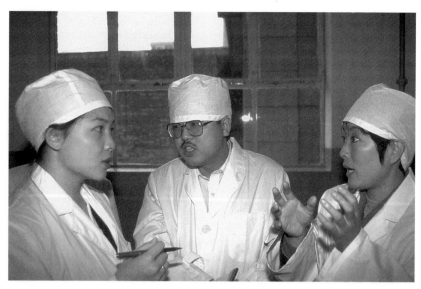

On factory inspection, Lanzhou

TAO REN WAN

Fructus Persica Pills
Peach Kernel Pills
Run Chang Wan
Master Shen's Book for Revering Life
(Shen Shi Zun Sheng Shu)
Dr. Shen Jin-Ao, 1773 A.D.

Caution: This is a very popular product and is commonly found in counterfeit form with several different names.

Common Usage: Laxative.

Description: Tao Ren Wan treats the problem of dry stool or constipation in the elderly or chronically sick whose bodies do not produce enough fluid to moisten the stool. This formula relieves the constitutional problem of a deficiency of body fluids and blood. Symptoms include a dry mouth, unquenchable thirst, dull skin, dull hair and nails, and constipation.

Chinese Diagnosis: Constipation can occur as a result of getting a common cold with a fever which has moved inward, invading the intestines and causing the stool to dry out and stagnate. Two herbs in this prescription help to deal with this condition. *Qiang Huo* (notopterygium rhizome) fights a common cold and expels the external sickness evil, and *Da Huang* (rhubarb root) clears heat from the intestines and purges the stool.

This formula should not be taken long term. If constipation is a chronic problem, please see a licensed healthcare provider.

Ingredients in the Formula:
Da Huang (rhubarb root) is the main purgative herb in Chinese Medicine. It cools internal heat which dries out essential body fluids necessary to moisten the stool, and purges accumulated feces in the intestines.

Hu Ma Ren (flax seed) and *Tao Ren* (peach kernel) are oily seeds which lubricate the intestines. They provide a mild laxative effect and work best with those who have weak constitutions—the elderly or those who are recovering from illness. Hu Ma Ren also helps replenish yin fluids which are essential in moistening the stool.

Dang Gui Wei (angelica sinensis root tails) nourishes blood which provides essential body fluids in the intestines.

Qiang Huo (notopterygium rhizome) expels wind and relieves a common cold.

Dosage: 4 pills three times per day.

TIAN MA WAN

Gastrodia Pills
Collected Treatises of Zhang Jing-Yue
(Jing Yue Quan Shu)
Dr. Zhang Jing-Yue, 1624 A.D.

Note: Many factories produce this product or similar products. I cannot vouch for the quality or effectiveness of products other than those produced by Lanzhou Foci Herb factory. As of this writing, I have not visited the factories that manufacture the other versions of this formula.

Common Usage: Arthritis, rheumatism, headache.

Description: This formula is very popular and variations of it are manufactured by many different companies with some alterations in the prescription. It is popular in China because it is designed to eliminate minor complaints of aches and pains. It is a general formula and includes herbs to treat neck and shoulder pain, low back pain, joint pain and pain caused by minor arthritis.

Chinese Diagnosis: Most neck, shoulder, back and knee pain is called "bi syndromes" or "wind damp bi pain." The herbs in this formula eliminate internal wind and dampness. Dampness creates stagnation and dull pain while wind makes the pain migrate from joint to joint and muscle to muscle.

Ingredients in the Formula:

Du Huo (angelica pubescens rhizome) and *Qiang Huo* (notopterygium rhizome) are paired herbs that eliminate wind damp bi pain. Du Huo focuses on the lower back, knees and legs, while Qiang Huo helps the neck and shoulders. They dry dampness and stop headache pain.

Shu Di Huang (prepared rehmannia root), *Xuan Shen* (scrophularia root) and *Dang Gui* (angelica sinensis root) balance the warm, drying qualities of many of the herbs in this formula by nourishing blood and body fluids which lubricate areas that needs moistening.

Du Zhong (eucommia bark) strengthens the liver and the kidneys, promotes proper circulation of blood, and can be taken for lower back pain, sore, weak knees, and frequent urination. It also lowers blood pressure.

Tian Ma (gastrodia rhizome) extinguishes internal wind, stops spasms and reduces irritability. Tian Ma is especially helpful in eliminating dizziness, headaches and pain.

Niu Xi (achyranthes root) strengthens the liver and kidneys, nourishes tendons and bones, and lowers blood pressure. It also directs energy downward away from the head.

Bi Xie (dioscorea hypoglauca rhizome) separates the pure from the impure, removing toxins and excess dampness. It softens tendons, relaxes muscles, and opens the meridians and channels especially to the lower back, legs, knees and feet.

Xiang Fu (cyperus rhizome) aids digestion and normalizes the liver which controls tendons. It moves stagnant Qi which when blocked can cause pain and discomfort.

Dosage: 8 pills three times per day.

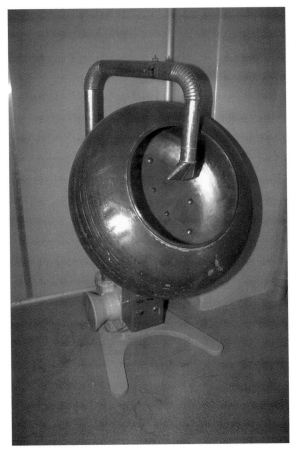

Drying pan, Lanzhou

TIAN WANG BU XIN DAN

Heaven King Tonify Heart Pills
Emperor Tea Pills
Secret Investigations into Obtaining Health
(She Sheng Mi Pou)
Dr. Hong Jiu-You, 1638 A.D.

Caution: This product is copied by many different factories. I have seen several different counterfeit versions.

Common Usage: Regulates and calms the heart and mind.

Description: This formula treats minor complaints associated with the heart—insomnia, palpitations, excessive dreaming or dream-disturbed sleep, forgetfulness, difficulty concentrating, burning urination, and mouth or tongue ulcers.

Chinese Diagnosis: The heart must be properly nourished by blood and cooled by essential body fluids. If the fluids do not cool the heart properly, it will become overactive, disturbing sleep and causing restlessness. The heart has to work very hard. If not properly nourished and cooled down, the heart overworks and can become excessively stimulated.

According to Western Medicine, symptoms such as forgetfulness, excessive dreaming and difficulty concentrating are considered to be psychosomatic mental problems; they are treated with tranquilizers and other medications which do not really address the causes of these conditions. In Chinese Medicine such problems are recognized as a physical malady which can be treated. The treatment consists of nourishing blood and body fluids, cooling the heart, and calming the mind.

In Chinese Medicine, this condition is called "kidney and heart not communicating." The kidneys must steam body fluids that can be transported upwards to cool the heart; the heart must direct its vitality and warmth downward to the kidneys in order to keep the vital life force fire alive and well. Both must cooperate in order to maintain harmony and balance.

Ingredients in the Formula:

Dang Shen (codonopsis root) strengthens the spleen Qi and increases the body's overall energy. If the digestion can be improved, more nutrients can be extracted from food and can be utilized by the body, making healthy blood which cools the heart. When digestion is healthy, other bodily functions remain healthy. Dang Shen also restores necessary yin body fluids.

Dan Shen (salvia root) is the main herb given to patients in China who are having heart problems. It invigorates blood so that it doesn't stagnate; it helps to dilate the coronary arteries so that blood can move smoothly through the heart muscle; it eliminates chest pain, and calms the restless mind; it cools the blood to calm the heart.

Xuan Shen (scrophularia root), *Mai Men Dong* (ophiopogonis tuber), *Sheng Di Huang* (raw rehmannia root), and *Tian Men Dong* (asparagus tuber) replenish essential body fluids, cool the blood and calm the restless spirit. Tian Men Dong strengthens the kidneys so that they can deliver water to cool the heart and to cool heat that causes irritability. Mai Men Dong cools internal body heat and replenishes lost fluids, restoring emotional harmony. Xuan Shen replenishes fluids in the mouth and throat, cools the blood and calms the restless spirit. Sheng Di Huang calms the heart and the mind as well as fortifies the kidneys.

Suan Zao Ren (zizyphus seed), *Bai Zi Ren* (biota seed) and *Yuan Zhi* (polygala root) all calm the emotions and relax the mind. Suan Zao Ren nourishes liver blood which supports the heart. Bai Zi Ren sedates the heart and calms the spirit. All three eliminate insomnia and restlessness.

Fu Ling (poria cocos fungus) normalizes proper fluid management in the body. It drains excess dampness from some areas where excess fluids don't belong and moves essential fluids to areas where they do belong. It also calms the heart and the mind.

Wu Wei Zi (schisandra fruit) stops excessive sweating and calms the spirit and the mind. Because of its astringent nature, it helps the body maintain homeostasis by controlling the loss of body fluids.

Dang Gui (angelica sinensis root) nourishes blood and helps the blood to flow properly. If blood moves too fast, it creates heat; if it moves too slowly, it causes stagnation. Dang Gui regulates the normal function of the movement of blood. When there is not enough blood, the heart has to work too hard and becomes overworked and may experience palpitations.

Jie Geng (platycodon root) directs the energy of the herbs upwards into the lungs where they can be directed to the heart.

Dosage: 8 pills three times per day.

XIANG FU LI ZHONG WAN

Regulate the Middle Pills
Discussion of Cold Induced Disorders
(Shang Han Lun)
Dr. Chang Chung-Ching, 142–220 A.D.

Common Usage: Severe abdominal and digestive problems.

Description: A variation of two formulas, Li Zhong Wan and Si Jun Zi Tang Wan (Four Gentlemen; see page 178), Xiang Fu Li Zhong Wan treats severe digestive difficulties associated with cold and dampness. This is referred to as spleen and stomach deficient and cold. In this situation, there is also kidney yang deficiency (a weakness of the life force fire).

The symptoms include severe abdominal cold, bloating, vomiting (often with a complete inability to keep food down), loose stools, no appetite, excessive clear saliva, cold hands and feet, slight sweating, chest and/or stomach pain, and weak, imperceptible pulse. Even more extreme symptoms include a lack of thirst, cold sweating, clear, watery diarrhea, and entire body cold.

Ingredients in the Formula:

Dang Shen (codonopsis root) raises deficient Qi, improves digestion and assists the lungs.

Bai Zhu (atractylodes rhizome) dries dampness that impedes digestion and warms the digestion.

Xiang Fu (cyperus rhizome) harmonizes digestion, eliminating pain and discomfort in the stomach and intestines.

Gan Jiang (dried ginger rhizome) warms the digestive fire, warms the middle of the body and warms the lungs to improve breathing.

Gan Cao (licorice root) harmonizes the formula, improves digestion and provides more energy.

Dosage: 8 pills three times per day.

XIANG SHA LIU JUN WAN

Xiang Fu and Sha Ren Six Gentlemen Tea Pills
Aplotaxis-Amomum Pills
Six Gentlemen Tea Pills
Comprehensive Medicine According to Master Zhang
(Zhang Shi Yi Tong)
Dr. Zhang Lu-Xuan, 1695 A.D.

Caution: I have seen counterfeit versions of this product.

Common Usage: Improves digestion, drains dampness.

Description: This is Four Gentlemen, plus four additional herbs which focus on tonifying and regulating digestion.

Chinese Diagnosis: This formula is designed to treat spleen deficiency (weak digestion) with associated dampness and cold. When excess fluid accumulates in the middle (spleen and stomach), it slows the normal flow of food and Qi, dulling the appetite and making digestion sluggish. When digestion is sluggish and there is dampness, the digestive fire is reduced. This causes an individual to eat very little and to feel overly full. Other symptoms are reduced appetite, nausea, belching, bloating and loose stool.

This is a good formula for morning sickness.

Ingredients in the Formula:

Dang Shen (codonopsis root), *Bai Zhu* (atractylodes rhizome), *Fu Ling* (poria cocos fungus), and *Gan Cao* (licorice root) improve digestive function, dry dampness and boost energy. Four Gentlemen also improves the immune system. Blood is manufactured by the body from the nutrients provided by the food that we eat. When our digestion is good, the body produces healthy blood which nourishes all the cells in our system. The immune system flourishes specifically through the production of more white blood cells, T cells and B cells, lymphocytes and platelets (which stop excessive bleeding).

Chen Pi (aged citrus peel) regulates the energy in the middle of the body and is drying, assisting the other herbs when there is dampness. It can eliminate bloating, belching, nausea and vomiting. It also clears phlegm (sticky dampness) from the lungs to improve breathing for patients who have shortness of breath, cough or long term nasal congestion without yellow mucus.

Sha Ren (amomum fruit) dries dampness, regulates digestion and stops vomiting. It is an excellent herb for morning sickness.

Ban Xia (pinellia rhizome) regulates middle Qi (spleen and stomach Qi), directing Qi downward when it has become stuck. It is the principal herb to clear phlegm which can create digestive sluggishness and a cough as well as many other complications.

Mu Xiang (saussurea root) stops vomiting, nausea, and bloating. It normalizes the function of the small and large intestine, stops diarrhea, and keeps the intestines from becoming sluggish.

Dosage: 8 pills two times per day.

XIANG SHA YANG WEI WAN

Auklandia and Amomum to Strengthen the Stomach Pills
Restoration of Health from the Myriad Diseases
(Wan Bing Hui Chun)
Dr. Gong Ting-Xian, 1587 A.D.

Common Usage: Aids digestion, stops bloating, drains dampness.

Description: This product is similar to Xiang Xia Liu Jun Wan (see above) but has even stronger actions to fortify digestion.

Description: One of the most common digestive problems is dampness which slows proper movement of Qi and restricts the normal function of digestion. Dampness is usually created by poor dietary habits such as drinking beverages with ice, eating cold, uncooked foods, and relying heavily on dairy products as a food source. Cold and dampness weaken the digestive process and contribute to a greater accumulation of dampness which affects the appetite.

Chinese Diagnosis: Xiang Sha Yang Wei Wan addresses this critical problem by strengthening the function of the spleen and stomach and by draining dampness. Symptoms of dampness affecting spleen and stomach include reduced or no appetite, loss of taste in the mouth, bloating after eating only a small amount of food, discomfort after eating and loose stool. If this continues long term, it can lead to fatigue, weakness, pale skin and generalized chronic listlessness.

Ingredients in the Formula:
This formula consists of *Four Gentlemen* (Si Jun Zi Tang Wan; see page 178) with the addition of *Chen Pi* (aged citrus peel), *Ban Xia* (pinellia rhizome), *Mu Xiang* (saussurea root) and *Sha Ren* (amomum fruit) (see Xiang Sha Liu Jun Zi Wan above).

Huo Xiang (patchouli herb) regulates dampness. This is different than draining dampness in that it regulates fluids. It may well be that an individual can have edema (too much fluid) in one area of the body and have dry skin at the same time. Enough fluids are present, but those fluids are unable to do their job properly. Huo Xiang directs them to the proper locations so that they can moisten and nourish rather than stagnate and cause bloating.

Xiang Fu (cyperus rhizome) regulates the liver which often interferes with digestion. The liver is said to become overactive when congested and to invade the stomach and spleen, blocking the natural downward flow of Qi. This causes energy to stagnate and Qi to be rebellious—to flow against the natural, normal direction or to flow in excess in the right direction. Rebellious Qi rises causing a regurgitation of food, belching and sometimes vomiting. Xiang Fu controls this rebellion of excess liver Qi.

Bai Dou Kou (cardamon fruit) regulates dampness, improves appetite, warms and sends digestive Qi downward in its proper direction. It eliminates bloating, nausea and vomiting.

Hou Po (magnolia bark) regulates dampness, normalizes the function of the bowels, and stops vomiting and diarrhea.

Zhi Shi (aurantium fruit) breaks up stagnation in the digestive tract, keeps food from becoming sluggish in the intestines and normalizes bowel function.

Dosage: 8 pills three times per day.

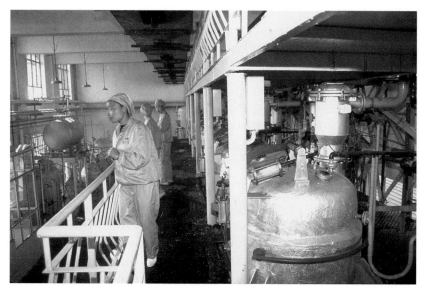

Herb cookers, Lanzhou

XIAO CHAI HU TANG WAN

Minor Bupleurum Formula Pills
Discussion of Cold-Induced Disorders
(Shang Han Lun)
Dr. Chang Chung-Ching, 142–220 A.D.

Caution: This is often found in counterfeit form.

Common Usage: Lingering common cold.

Description: This prescription treats a common cold which does not improve and is starting to invade deeper layers of the body. It is the second stage of the common cold, called Shao Yang syndrome. Dr. Chang observed that a common cold can evolve through six stages. If a cold worsens into the third stage, it will invade the interior and attack the lungs or the intestines, the Yang Ming level. Shao Yang Level is the second stage where the disease is trapped between the exterior and the interior.

Symptoms include alternating fever and chills, an internal struggle between the body and the disease as the disease tries to penetrate more deeply. It is accompanied by a dry throat, bitter taste in the mouth, dizziness, irritability, bloated chest, shallow breathing, low appetite, nausea and perhaps vomiting.

Based on the symptoms, it can be seen that the disease is beginning to affect the digestion (nausea, low appetite) and the lungs (difficult breathing). This formula also can be taken when a woman gets a common cold during menses. The Chinese teach that taking very strong cold-fighting herbs during menses is potentially damaging to women because they are more vulnerable at this time. The Chinese say that the House of Blood (uterus and associated meridians) is open during menses and therefore makes women more susceptible to the affects of strong, cold herbs.

This prescription follows the harmonizing principle of treating disease: a balance between strengthening the body's resistance and fighting infection. Other approaches include the sweating method, which is used in the first stage of a cold, or the heat clearing method, which would be used for disease that has completely invaded the interior.

Ingredients in the Formula:

Chai Hu (bupleurum root) specifically treats sickness that is trapped between the exterior and the interior (otherwise known as Shao Yang Syndrome). It also helps to relieve a fever, and is anti-inflammatory, antibacterial and antiviral.

Huang Qin (scutellaria root) reduces fever in the upper part of the body including the chest, neck and head, as well as in the stomach and in the intestines. It fights infections because of its antibiotic properties.

Ban Xia (pinellia rhizome) clears phlegm and dampness to protect the lungs, harmonizes the digestive system and normalizes the middle.

Sheng Jiang (fresh ginger rhizome) warms the digestive system to relieve nausea, poor appetite, and to balance the effects of cold herbs on the stomach. It can also dissolve phlegm.

Dang Shen (codonopsis root) builds the immune system, assists the digestion and nourishes the normal energy of the body so that it can better resist sickness. It also strengthens the lungs which are considered the be the sensitive organ, most easily susceptible to sickness.

Da Zao (black jujube date) harmonizes the digestion and builds energy.

Gan Cao (licorice root) harmonizes the actions of the other herbs and aids digestion.

Dosage: 8 pills three times per day.

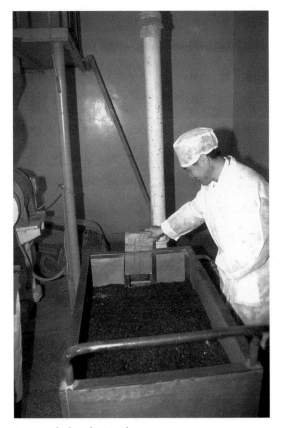

Inspecting herb quality, Lanzhou

XIAO YAO WAN

Free and Easy Rambling Pills
Relaxed Wanderer
Free and Easy Wanderer
Imperial Grace Formulary of the Tai Ping Era
(Tai Ping Hui Min He Ji Ju Fang)
Imperial Medical Department, 1078–1085 A.D.

Caution: This is the most popular Chinese product available in the U.S. I have seen many counterfeit versions of it. In counterfeit form, it is sometimes called Hsiao Yao Wan. There are many other versions of this product which are produced by American companies and are more expensive than this Chinese product.

Common Usage: PMS, stress, anemia.

Description: A popular patent medicine in the United States, Xiao Yao Wan is often taken by women between the menses to eliminate the symptoms of PMS. These symptoms occur because of concurrent stagnant liver Qi and blood deficiency. Xiao Yao Wan enriches blood and helps regulate the liver which controls the movement of Qi and blood in the body.

Chinese Diagnosis: The emotional symptoms of PMS—distress, upset and anxiety—are commonly looked upon by Western doctors as being psychosomatic, but according to Chinese Medical theory, they are very real, physical symptoms. Other symptoms of PMS include bloating, fatigue, headache, dizziness, blurry vision, dry mouth and throat, as well as reduced appetite and an irregular menstrual cycle, including cramps. Many of these symptoms can be relieved by regular consumption of Xiao Yao Wan.

If a woman loses too much blood from menstrual bleeding and her body can't replace it, normal function of the organs will be adversely affected, causing depression and other emotional reactions. The liver is most commonly affected and liver constriction often occurs, leading to pain and discomfort. Such discomfort can show up as headaches, a tight, uncomfortable chest, or digestive complications including diarrhea or constipation as well as more obvious uterine cramping.

Ingredients in the Formula:

Chai Hu (bupleurum root) relieves Qi stagnation in the liver (constriction of emotions) and alleviates disharmony of the chest and stomach, controlling such symptoms as bloating, nausea and indigestion.

Bai Shao (white peony root) builds blood and relaxes the liver. This is extremely important for normal menstruation because the liver controls the flow of blood and Qi in the body. If there is stagnation from stress or other reasons, the blood and Qi will not flow easily and menstruation will be difficult.

Dang Gui (angelica sinensis root) builds and regulates blood and, most importantly, controls contractions of the uterus, stopping cramps. Dang Gui is the single most important herb in gynecology because it helps balance and harmonize the female organs.

Bai Zhu (atractylodes rhizome) improves digestion and assimilation of nutrients and thus helps to build healthier blood.

Bo He (mint herb) calms the emotions and addresses gynecological problems by soothing the liver and eliminating constraint brought about by stress.

Fu Ling (poria cocos fungus) improves digestion and drains excess fluids. It is very common for women to retain fluids just before their menses, and Fu Ling promotes urination to drain excess dampness. It also helps the other herbs to calm the emotions.

Gan Cao (licorice root) harmonizes the formula, improving digestion and lung function.

Sheng Jiang (fresh ginger rhizome) harmonizes digestion and warms the middle.

Dosage: 8 pills three times per day.

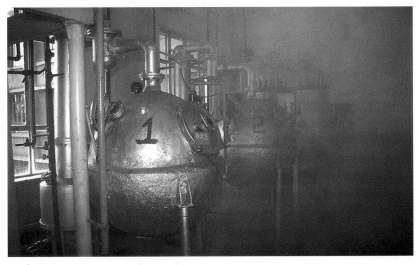

Lanzhou Foci Factory

YANG RONG WAN

Promote Health Pills
[Based on: Ren Shen Yang Rong Wan]
Ginseng Promote Health Pills
Imperial Grace Formulary of the Tai Ping Era
(Tai Ping Hui Min He Ji Ju Fang)
Imperial Medical Department, 1078–1085 A.D.

Special Warning: If you are pregnant, do not take this formula without first consulting a licensed practitioner.

Common Usage: Easy bruising, spotting between periods, spotting when pregnant.

Description: Yang Rong Wan treats conditions of excessive menstrual bleeding. These conditions include spotting between periods, bleeding long after menses should have stopped or spotting when pregnant. This is generally caused by a deficiency of Qi and by weak blood vessels which are unable to contain blood.

This formula nourishes blood, improves digestion to make more blood, and promotes energy. It also strengthens the kidneys and helps to nourish body fluids which are essential in the manufacture of blood. Blood deficiency is more significant than anemia because it may affect other components of blood such as white blood cells. It is also possible when someone is blood deficient that they may not have enough platelets. Since platelets coagulate to stop bleeding, they are essential in preventing excessive blood loss.

The classic formula is called Jiao Ai Tang, (Donkey-hide Gelatin and Mugwort Formula). It contains Si Wu Tang Wan, plus E Jiao (Donkey-hide gelatin) and Ai Ye (Chinese mugwort).

Symptoms include spotting between periods, post-partum bleeding, pale face, pale skin, small, short periods with pale, thin blood without clots, fatigue, easy bruising, a pale tongue or a period that continues for a week or longer.

Ingredients in the Formula:

Si Wu Tang Wan (Four Substances; see page 179) nourishes blood and promotes normal circulation, regulates the menstrual cycle, and stops cramps and pain. The four ingredients are:

Dang Gui (angelica sinensis root) nourishes and regulates blood. It is important in assisting women both with hormones and with blood.

Shu Di Huang (prepared rehmannia root) nourishes blood to eliminate anemia. It also helps replenish yin body fluids which include hormones.

Bai Shao (white peony root) nourishes blood, stops pain, cramps and spasms. It helps to eliminate cramps by promoting the production of more blood and by helping the body to retain vital fluids which lubricate muscles, tendons and bones. Bai Shao is also an important herb to help normalize the liver function which controls blood flow during the menstrual cycle.

Chuan Xiong (ligusticum root) regulates blood, and helps stop pain, cramps and headache. It is a very important gynecological herb.

Ai Ye (artemesia herb; Chinese mugwort) stops bleeding, warms the womb and eliminates infertility. Taken internally, it stops prolonged menstrual bleeding and cramps. It is known to calm a restless fetus.

E Jiao (donkey-hide gelatin) nourishes blood and stops bleeding, especially heavy menstrual bleeding or uterine bleeding. It also produces more yin fluids which include the normal production of hormones. Hormones are necessary to maintain homeostasis, harmony and balance of body functions.

Yi Mu Cao (leonurus herb; motherwort) translates as "benefit the mother grass." It normalizes menstrual difficulties, stops PMS pain, alleviates post-partum pain and helps to improve energy. It also helps break up cysts and fibroids.

Du Zhong (eucommia bark) strengthens the liver and the kidneys, promotes proper circulation of blood and calms the restless fetus. It can be taken for low back pain, sore, weak knees and frequent urination. It also lowers blood pressure. All of these are common problems for women during their pregnancy.

Mai Men Dong (ophiopogonis tuber) nourishes yin body fluids which are necessary in order to produce sufficient blood.

Huang Qi (astragalus root) and *Bai Zhu* (atractylodes rhizome) enhance overall energy by improving digestion. Huang Qi also has a lifting effect to protect against miscarriage.

Chen Pi (aged citrus peel) and *Xiang Fu* (cyperus rhizome) regulate middle Qi and improve digestion. When digestion improves, the body manufactures more blood and maintains harmony more easily.

Sha Ren (amomum fruit) helps digestion by eliminating excessive dampness which slows down healthy digestive function. It also calms the fetus.

Xiang Fu (cyperus rhizome) harmonizes digestion and relieves menstrual difficulties, including irregular menses, cramping and discomfort.

Fu Ling (poria cocos fungus) drains excess fluids and improves digestion as well as calms the mind.

Dosage: 8 pills three times per day.

YANG YING WAN

Ginseng Tonic Pills
[Based on: Ren Shen Yang Ying Wan]
Ren Shen Tonify Yin and Yang Pills
Imperial Grace Formulary of the Tai Ping Era
(Tai Ping Hui Min He Ji Ju Fang)
Imperial Medical Department, 1078–1085 A.D.

Common Usage: Chronic illness, fatigue, weakness.

Description: This formula is designed to build energy and vitality. It contains herbs to build Qi, warm the interior of the body, and elevate vital energy.

Ingredients in the Formula:

Shu Di Huang (prepared rehmannia root), *Bai Shao* (white peony root), and *Dang Gui* (angelica sinensis root) promote the building of blood.

Dang Shen (codonopsis root), *Bai Zhu* (atractylodes rhizome), *Huang Qi* (astragalus root), *Fu Ling* (poria cocos fungus), and *Gan Cao* (licorice root) work together to produce more Qi in the body and to improve digestion. In Chinese Medicine, the foundation of many formulas is an herbal prescription to improve digestion, which is considered to be the key to good health.

Rou Gui (cinnamon bark) warms and strengthens the body at the deepest level of vitality. It also supports the other herbs in the formula as they nourish blood and Qi.

Chen Pi (aged citrus peel) regulates Qi and keeps the energy moving in the body. It also helps to regulate digestion.

Da Zao (black jujube dates) harmonizes digestion and helps promote energy.

Sheng Jiang (fresh ginger rhizome) warms the middle and improves digestion.

Wu Wei Zi (schisandra fruit) and *Yuan Zhi* (polygala root) calm the mind.

Dosage: 8 pills three times per day.

YIN CHIAO JIE DU WAN

Yin Qiao Chieh Tu Pian
Honeysuckle and Forsythia Clear Toxins Pills
[Based on: Yin Qiao San]
[Honeysuckle and Forsythia Powder]
Systematic Differentiation of Warm Diseases
(Wen Bing Tiao Bian)
Dr. Wu Ju-Tong, 1798 A.D.

Note: This is one of the most popular herbal products in the U.S. because it is so effective in treating the common cold. Many factories manufacture this product, and it is available from many different sources. Plum Flower Brand has at least two products by this name which are listed in the back of this book. Other versions of this formula may contain drugs and food coloring. There are also many counterfeit versions of this product.

Common Usage: Common cold, sore throat.

Description: Yin Qiao San is one of the classic formulas for treating common cold. It is taken for what the Chinese call "wind-heat," a common cold with fever, sore throat, nasal congestion and yellow mucus.

It should be differentiated from other types of common cold, such as "wind-cold," "wind-damp" and summer heat (stomach flu) which should be treated with other formulas.

Chinese Diagnosis: With a wind-heat condition, look for heat signs such as fever with little or no chills, slight sweating, thirst, headache and a sore, scratchy throat. A Chinese doctor would feel a floating, superficial pulse because the protective energy (Wei Qi) of the body is moving toward the surface of the skin layer in order to repel the invasion of wind evil (pathogenic bacteria). Wind evil is said to invade through the pores of the skin.

It is best to take this formula at the earliest stages of a common cold. Look for the first sign of sickness which is usually unexplained fatigue. Your body is already fighting the cold by mustering your reserve energy in order to combat the invasion of pathogens such as bacteria or a virus.

Ingredients in the Formula:
Jin Yin Hua (lonicera; honeysuckle flower) and *Lian Qiao* (forsythia fruit) are the two main herbs in this formula. They clear heat and reduce swelling which often accompany a sore throat. They also have anti-bacterial qualities which make them especially effective in fighting colds.

Niu Bang Zi (burdock; arctium seed) clears wind-heat, reduces swelling and helps relieve a sore throat. It helps to open pores, causing a sweat which breaks the fever.

Bo He (mint herb) clears heat especially in the throat and head. It relieves sore throat and headache and clears heat from the face and eyes. It also causes a sweat to reduce a fever.

Jie Geng (platycodon root) directs the energy of the herbs upward to the lungs and throat. It assists digestion, strengthens the lungs which control the protective energy of the body (wei Qi) and improves resistance to disease.

Jing Jie (schizonepeta herb) can be used in any type of common cold. It induces the body to sweat, opening the pores and driving out the cause of this illness. It also has anti-viral and anti-bacterial properties.

Dan Zhu Ye (bamboo leaf; lophatherum herb) cools heat and helps calm irritability when someone is sick. It also soothes the throat and clears sores from the mouth and tongue.

Dan Dou Chi (prepared soybean) treats both wind-heat and wind-cold and helps to calm irritability which is often associated with fever and illness.

Gan Cao (licorice root) harmonizes the formula and helps to direct the energy of the herbs wherever they are most needed in the body.

Dosage: 8 pills three times per day.

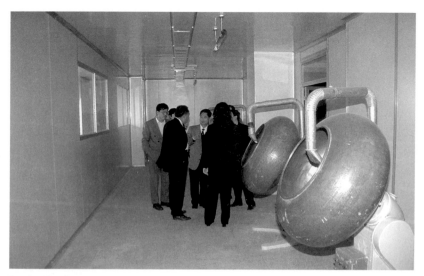

Lanzhou Foci Factory

YU DAI WAN

Stop Leukorrhea Pills
Standards for Diagnosis and Treatment
(Zheng Zhi Zhun Sheng)
Dr. Wang Ken-Tang, 1602 A.D.

Common Usage: Stops vaginal discharge.

Description: This prescription treats damp heat in the lower burner (kidney, urinary bladder, large intestine, small intestine, sexual organs). In this instance, dampness and heat have collected in the area around the uterus and female organs. Heat and dampness create a type of inflammation which forces out accumulated body fluids. It is often associated with internal heat in the blood and bloody vaginal discharge. The discharge should have a yellow color; there could be associated itching, pain and/or strong smell.

Other symptoms might include burning urination, lower abdominal pain, a bitter taste in the mouth and dry throat.

Ingredients in the Formula:

Chun Gen Pi (ailanthus root bark) clears heat and dampness, especially in the lower abdomen. It is astringent, stopping the discharge of fluids.

Huang Bai (phellodendron bark) clears heat and dampness from the lower abdomen, uterus and genitals.

Gao Liang Jiang (galanga rhizome) stops pain in the middle and lower part of the abdomen and balances the cold properties of the other herbs.

Si Wu Tang (Four Substances; see page 179) nourishes and invigorates blood to support the normal function of a woman's body. Only when the body is properly nourished can it heal itself and rid itself of symptoms such as vaginal discharge.

Dang Gui (angelica sinensis root) nourishes and regulates blood. It is important in assisting women both with hormones and with blood.

Shu Di Huang (prepared rehmannia root) nourishes blood to eliminate anemia. It also helps replenish yin body fluids which include hormones.

Bai Shao (white peony root) nourishes blood, stops pain, cramps and spasms. It helps to eliminate cramps by promoting the production of more blood and by helping the body to retain vital fluids which lubricate muscles, tendons and bones. Bai Shao is also an important herb to help normalize the liver function which controls blood flow during the menstrual cycle.

Chuan Xiong (ligusticum root) regulates blood, and helps stop pain, cramps and headache. It is a very important gynecological herb.

Dosage: 8 pills three times per day.

ZHI BAI DI HUANG WAN

Anemarrhena, Phellodendron and Rehmannia Pills
Zhi Bai Ba Wei Wan
Anemarrhena and Phellodendron Eight Flavor Tea Pills
Pattern, Cause, Pulse, and Treatment
(Zheng Yin Mai Zhi)
Dr. Qin Jing-Ming, 1702 A.D.

Caution: This is one of the most popular products in China. It is widely found in counterfeit form. I have seen it called Chih Bai Di Huang Wan, Chin Pai Di Huang Wan, Chih Pai Di Huang Wan, as well as other names.

Common Usage: Nightsweats, hot flashes, menopause.

Description: This is a very popular formula, especially for menopausal women. One of the most common causes of menopausal symptoms such as night sweats and hot flashes is liver and kidney yin deficiency plus heat signs.

Chinese Diagnosis: When the yin is insufficient, it allows the complimentary yang (heat) to rise, causing hot flashes or night sweats. Body fluids are yin. When there is not enough fluid to control heat, fire rises out of control. The heat escapes to the surface of the skin, opening the pores and causing a sweat.

Ingredients in the Formula:
The foundation of this formula is *Liu Wei Di Huang Wan* (Six Flavor Rehmannia Tea Pills; see page 85) which treats Kidney yin deficiency. The following six herbs nourish Yin fluids and strengthen the kidney function.

Shan Zhu Yu (cornus fruit) strengthens kidney function, stops excessive urination and preserves vital fluids.

Shan Yao (dioscorea root) improves digestion and appetite, assists weak lungs, and nourishes the kidneys.

Shu Di Huang (prepared rehmannia root) nourishes blood, Yin and Jing. It also assists the heart and the liver which require an abundance of blood in order to function normally.

Fu Ling (poria cocos fungus) strengthens digestion and regulates vital fluids in the body.

Mu Dan Pi (moutan peony root bark) cools the blood and clears heat in the liver which burns up yin fluids.

Ze Xie (alisma rhizome) clears heat from the kidneys which burns up yin fluids and drains excess dampness.

This variation of the formula adds *Zhi Mu* (anemarrhena rhizome) and *Huang Bai* (phellodendron bark) to reduce heat and nourish yin. Both of the additional herbs are cold and thus clear heat.

Dosage: 8 pills three times per day.

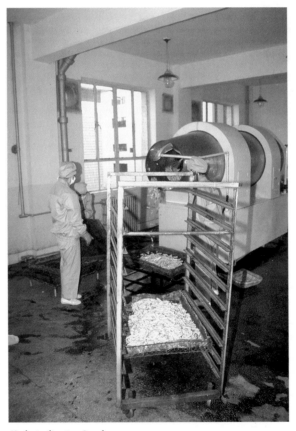

Herb sterilization, Lanzhou

ZI SHENG WAN

Promote Life Pills
[Based on: Si Jun Zi Tang]
Four Gentlemen Formula
Imperial Grace Formulary of the Tai Ping Era
(Tai Ping Hui Min He Ji Ju Fang)
Imperial Medical Department, 1078–1085 A.D.

Common Usage: Improves digestion.

Description: Zi Sheng Wan is a broad spectrum, complete and balanced formula to cover a wide range of digestive difficulties. As suggested by the translation of the name, Zi Sheng Wan improves the quality of life by improving digestion.

It addresses problems of loose stool, low appetite, gas, nausea, abdominal pain, malabsorption of food, belching, bloating and the feeling of fullness after eating. It can be taken long term by anyone with these digestive problems.

A good look through any one of the many large chain drug stores will show you that digestive complaints are a major problem in this society. Massive amounts of shelf space are devoted to products designed to remedy stomach problems. None of the products offered in drug stores does anything more than to provide temporary relief from minor complaints; Chinese Medicine, on the other hand, offers formulas which not only eliminate the minor short term complaints but also fortify and improve digestion.

Chinese Diagnosis: Zi Sheng Wan addresses a broad spectrum of digestive problems. In addition, it supports the function of the kidneys which store the vital life force energy, strengthens the lungs to improve breathing, and calms the heart and spirit when someone is anxious. It can also work to prevent colds and flu, bolstering the immune system to fight off invasions of bacteria and viruses.

Ingredients in the Formula:

Dang Shen (codonopsis root), *Bai Zhu* (atractylodes rhizome), *Fu Ling* (poria cocos fungus), and *Gan Cao* (licorice root) improve digestive function, dry dampness and boost energy. Four Gentlemen also improves the immune system. Blood is manufactured by the body from the nutrients provided by the food that we eat. When our digestion is good, the body produces healthy blood which nourishes all the cells in our system.

Yi Yi Ren (coix seed), *Bai Bian Dou* (dolichoris seed) and *Bai Dou Kou* (cardamon seed) drain dampness and strengthen digestion. When the digestive system is overwhelmed by cold damp foods, such as icy drinks and dairy products, it becomes sluggish and the body cannot properly process the dampness. This dampness eventually becomes phlegm and collects in the nasal passages, sinuses and lungs.

Ju Hong (orange peel) regulates the energy in the stomach and is drying, assisting other herbs to drain excess dampness which stagnates in the intestines. It can reduce belching, nausea, and vomiting. It can also help clear phlegm from the sinuses and lungs to improve breathing.

Shen Qu (fermented leaven), *Shan Zha* (hawthorn fruit) and *Mai Ya* (sprouted barley) prevent food from stagnating in the stomach and reduce the accumulation of fats and cholesterol in the digestive system. They also prevent that feeling of food being stuck in the stomach, causing bloating, belching and gas.

Qian Shi (euryale seed) and *Shan Yao* (dioscorea root) strengthen the kidney function and improve digestion. In Chinese Medicine, vital life force energy derives from two sources—the kidneys and the spleen. It is said that "pre-heaven" (congenital) Qi is stored in the kidneys and "post-heaven" Qi is derived from the spleen which extracts it from the food we eat. Qian Shi helps the body store that vital life force essence and strengthen digestion which replaces the essence that is lost through day-to-day living. Shan Yao strengthens both kidneys and spleen, improving digestion and supporting the kidneys.

Lian Zi (lotus seed) improves digestion and helps the body retain vital life force energy. It stops chronic diarrhea and can calm the spirit, relieving anxiety.

Huo Xiang (patchouli herb) regulates dampness. This is different than draining dampness in that it moves fluids to areas where they are lacking. It may well be that an individual can have edema (too much fluid) in one area of the body and still have dry skin. That indicates that enough fluids are present, but they are unable to do their job properly. It can also help to prevent common colds and other illnesses such as influenza.

Jie Geng (platycodon root) improves digestion and helps to regulate the normal function of Qi. It can also strengthen the lungs, both to improve breathing and to promote the immune system.

Huang Lian (coptis rhizome) kills bacteria that could affect digestion. It is also known to calm the over-anxious heart.

Dosage: 8 pills two times per day.

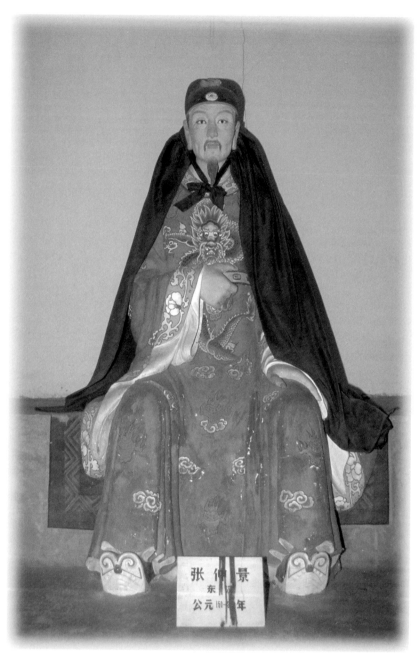

Dr. Chang Chung-Ching (142–220 A.D.)

6

PLUM FLOWER
CLASSIC FORMULAS

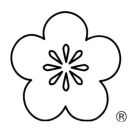

Plum Flower Classic Formulas are based on time-tested, historical formulas, many of which have been used effectively for thousands of years. Many of these formulas are now available in pill form for the first time. Until recently, these prescriptions were found only in the pharmacies of herbal doctors.

Every product in this line is manufactured by well-known factories in China which are certified GMP by an internationally recognized certification organization such as the Australian Therapeutic Goods Administration. Each of the following products is guaranteed to be 100% natural and to be completely free of pharmaceutical drugs and synthetic colors. No Plum Flower Brand product contains any mysterious, secret ingredients.

As I mentioned earlier in this book, the traditional method of preparing herbs in China is to cook them together like an herbal soup. It is this cooking process that makes Plum Flower formulas unique. They are prepared by a complex, low-temperature process that protects the integrity of the product while preserving all the active ingredients, including the volatile oils. All Plum Flower Brand products are scientifically tested in the factory to ensure that they are produced to the high standards of that factory. Plum Flower Brand products are also

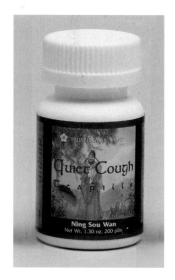

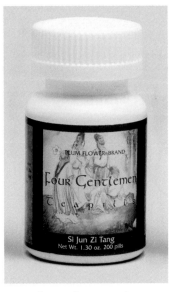

tested in independent third-party laboratories in order to ensure quality.

Some less reputable factories skip necessary steps in the manufacturing process in order to produce a cheaper product. Some use high heat extraction which is faster and therefore less expensive, but which damages the medicinal value of the herbs. Some manufacturers use cheap, low-grade herbs to reduce costs. Very often, such factories are not licensed, remain uninspected and do not comply with health and safety codes. Herbal products produced by these unlicensed factories are of dubious value and may potentially be dangerous.

Western herbal manufacturers of Chinese products usually grind up raw herbs and press them into tablets. My concern about these products is that they are not cooked; it is the cooking process that makes the raw herbs effective and easier to assimilate. Human beings are not herbivores (animals that can eat raw plants, digest cellulose and extract the vital essence from them). Over the centuries, Chinese doctors have learned that human beings are much healthier when they eat cooked food. They have also learned that patients recover more quickly from illness and are restored to health more readily when they consume properly prepared and cooked herbal formulas.

It is for these reasons that I have included Plum Flower Classic Formulas in this book. To my knowledge, these products are superior to any other Chinese herbal formulas available in the marketplace today.

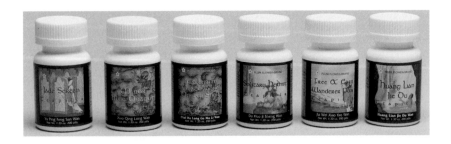

AN SHUI WAN

Peaceful Sleep Pills
[Based on: Suan Zao Ren Tang]
(Ziziphus Formula)
Essentials from the Golden Cabinet
(Jin Gui Yao Lue)
Dr. Chang Chung-Ching, 142–220 A.D.

Common Usage: Insomnia.

Description: An Shui Wan reduces mental agitation and restlessness, calming the mind to encourage sleep. It is a natural tranquilizer that relaxes and sedates the mind so that the individual may fall asleep easily and stay asleep.

An Sui Wan, unlike tranquilizing drugs, has no negative side effects and does not cause a hangover or drowsiness the next day. Nonetheless, caution is always advised when taking anything that might encourage drowsiness, especially when operating any type of machinery.

Chinese Diagnosis: Insomnia has two main causes. The first is a deficiency of liver blood which does not properly nourish the heart. The other cause is an uprising of heat caused by a deficiency of yin body fluids. In Chinese Medicine, Yin body fluids keep body heat in check. If those essential fluids are deficient, internal body heat will rise and disturb the mind, keeping an individual awake. An Shui Wan addresses these problems, both directly and indirectly, by improving digestion (which nourishes heart blood and liver blood) and by including herbs which tonify yin fluids to cool the heart.

Ingredients in the Formula:
Suan Zao Ren (zizyphus seed) nourishes the heart, feeds liver blood to support the heart, and calms the spirit.

Bai Zi Ren (biota seed) nourishes heart blood and quiets the mind, relieving anxiety, irritability and insomnia.

Yuan Zhi (polygala root) calms the heart and unblocks the coronary arteries and the heart channels to allow free flow of Qi and blood which cool the heart and properly nourish the heart muscle.

An Shui Wan also contains *Si Jun Zi Tang* (Four Gentlemen; see page 178), the main formula for improving digestion. When the digestion is working properly, the body produces enough blood to calm the heart and properly nourish all internal organs.

Chen Pi (aged citrus peel) regulates digestive Qi, promoting normal functioning of digestive energy, dries dampness which impedes proper digestion and prevents digestive sluggishness.

Shan Yao (dioscorea root) aids digestion and strengthens the kidneys which support both the liver and the heart.

Jie Geng (platycodon root) improves digestion and directs vital nutrients to the lungs so that they can be dispersed throughout the body.

Dang Gui (angelica sinensis root) helps to build blood and encourages the free flow of blood in the body.

Shi Chang Pu (acorus rhizome) opens orifices to improve smooth blood flow in the arteries and blood vessels.

Mai Men Dong (ophiopogonis tuber) clears heat from the heart and reduces irritability.

Wu Wei Zi (schisandra fruit) calms the spirit, quiets the heart and helps the heart contain its energy.

Xuan Shen (scrophularia root) and *Shu Di Huang* (prepared rehmannia root) clear heat, cool and nourish blood to calm the mind. By producing fluids, this formula cools heat in the heart and encourages sleep. Whenever there is excess heat in the body, restlessness and irritability will present themselves along with insomnia.

Han Fang Ji (stephania root) has anti-inflammatory qualities to reduce swelling and allow a better flow of energy in the body.

Jin Bu Huan (stephania sinica) is a strong herbal sedative, relaxing the mind and encouraging the eyes to close.

Dosage: 2 pills as needed.

BA JI YIN YANG WAN

Morinda Root Yin and Yang Pills
Modern Formula

Common Usage: Slows the aging process, restores energy.

Description: This is a formula designed to fortify both kidney yin and yang. In Chinese Medicine, the kidneys are considered the foundation of all energy. Source Qi, or Original Qi which is stored in the kidneys, is the genetic essence of the parents.

As people reach middle age, their kidney Qi starts to decline and they begin to show signs of aging. Symptoms of diminishing Qi include menopause, weakening vision, sore back and knees, impotence, incontinence, frequent urination or night time urination, forgetfulness, dementia and other typically age-related conditions. Because of our modern, fast-paced lifestyle, kidney yin (essential life force essence) is also depleted. It literally burns itself out due to over activity and destructive habits. These habits include a poor diet, being continually "on the run," drinking alcohol, taking prescription and recreational drugs, and failure to exercise. It is said by Chinese doctors that as people age, they begin to "dry out."

This formula replenishes the fire of life and the vital life force fluids that keep that fire under control and in harmony.

Ingredients in the Formula:

Ba Ji Tian (morinda root) and *Yin Yang Huo* (epimedium leaf) fortify kidney yang, strengthen bones, tendons and muscles.

Sheng Di Huang (raw rehmannia root) fortifies kidney yin and replenishes necessary body fluids.

Bi Xie (dioscorea hypoclauca rhizome) controls dampness, separating the pure from the impure. This is an important concept in Chinese Medicine, for the kidneys when properly functioning are said to separate the "good from the bad." In other words, they recycle proteins and other beneficial nutrients in the body and excrete waste materials. When the kidneys are healthy and functioning properly, the efficiency of the body is much greater. When kidney function wanes, the aging process kicks in, due in great part to the ineffective removal of waste products from the body.

Bai Shao (white peony root) nourishes blood and prevents excessive loss of fluids.

Jin Ying Zi (rosa laevigata fruit) prevents the loss of body fluids and fortifies the kidneys and their ability to retain the life force essence.

Xu Duan (dipsacus root) and *Gou Ji* (barometz rhizome) support the kidneys and liver, and strengthen the back, especially the lower back. They promote the movement of blood to prevent stiffness and debility. As people age, they tend to get less exercise; bodily processes slow down and people lose their flexibility.

Gou Qi Zi (lycium fruit) fortifies both kidney Yin and Yang, nourishes blood and retains the kidney life force essence.

Du Zhong (eucommia bark) fortifies the kidneys and liver and help to move blood and Qi, preventing stagnation. It strengthens the back, knees, tendons and bones.

Lian Zi (lotus seed) strengthens digestion and assists in the retention of the kidney life force essence.

Shan Zhu Yu (cornus fruit) fortifies the kidneys and helps retain the life force essence.

Dang Gui (angelica sinensis root) nourishes blood and moves blood to prevent stagnation.

Dosage: 8 pills three times per day.

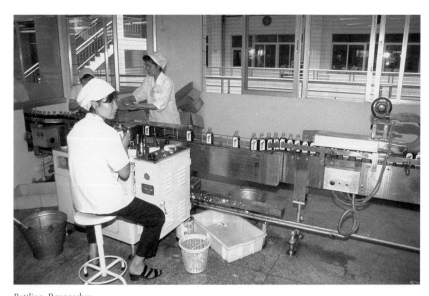

Bottling, Pangaoshou

BA ZHENG SAN

Eight Herb Powder to Rectify Urination
Eight Righteous Tea Pills
Imperial Grace Formulary of the Tai Ping Era
(Tai Ping Hui Min He Ji Ju Fang)
Imperial Medical Department, 1078–1085 A.D.

Common Usage: Urinary tract infection, bladder infections, kidney stones.

Description: Relieves urinary tract infection (UTI), especially UTI accompanied by burning, frequent urination, difficult, painful urination with bleeding, lower abdominal pain, dry mouth and throat. Can also be used for kidney stones which are not too large.

Chinese Diagnosis: This is considered lower burner damp heat or heat and dampness congealing in the lower burner. The lower burner is considered to be the area below the navel, the abode of the kidneys and urinary bladder. There are many causes for kidney or bladder infections, but a diet heavy in sweet, spicy-hot, rich foods and/or over-consumption of alcohol can lead to a predisposition to these conditions. There are several types of urinary tract infections (called lin) in Chinese Medicine, among them heat lin (hot, burning urinary tract infection), blood lin (blood in the urine) and stone lin (kidney stones).

Ingredients in the Formula:
Jin Qian Cao (lysimachia herb) promotes urination, expels stones and relieves painful, difficult urination.

Huang Bai (phellodendron bark) clears damp and heat from the lower burner (urinary bladder and kidney).

Mu Tong (akebia stem) promotes urination, clears damp heat, draining heat through the small intestine and bladder.

Qu Mai (dianthus herb) clears damp heat and relieves painful and difficult urination. It is especially effective with blood in the urine.

Bian Xu (polygonum herb) clears damp heat and promotes urination.

Che Qian Zi (plantago seed) treats any type of urinary problem, especially damp heat in the liver and lower burner.

Zhi Zi (gardenia fruit) clears damp heat from the liver and lower burner, cools blood and stops bleeding.

Da Huang (rhubarb root) clears heat and dampness from the lower part of the body. It also directs energy downward and out of the body.

Gan Cao (licorice root) harmonizes the formula.

Dosage: 8 pills three times per day.

BAN XIA HOU PO WAN

Pinellia and Magnolia Pills
Essentials from the Golden Cabinet
(Jin Gui Yao Lue)
Dr. Chang Chung-Ching, 142–220 A.D.

Special Warning: When using this formula, please be certain that there is no physical blockage in the throat. If the problem continues or worsens, please see a doctor.

Common Usage: Constricted throat, discomfort swallowing.

Description: Ban Xia Hou Po Wan addresses a problem which is considered psychosomatic in Western treatment. It is the sensation of having something stuck in the throat, of not being able to swallow, but for which there is no apparent physical cause. This simply means that there is no literal physical blockage that can be seen on an X-ray or MRI, but the individual feels something stuck in the throat.

Chinese Diagnosis: This is called "plum pit throat," a constriction in the throat with an inability to breathe deeply or a feeling of bloating in either the chest or the stomach. It is often caused by an emotional situation that the patient cannot figuratively "swallow." While there is an emotional cause for this condition, it is a physical reality from the Chinese medical perspective—Qi and phlegm knotted in the throat.

Ingredients in the Formula:

Ban Xia (pinellia rhizome) dissolves phlegm and releases stagnant Qi and phlegm which are stuck in the throat. Ban Xia dissolves the phlegm and helps to move Qi downward so that it doesn't remain stuck in the throat.

Hou Po (magnolia bark) transforms stagnant phlegm and dampness, helps the digestive process remove fluids and phlegm, and moves Qi downward to open the throat and the chest.

Fu Ling (poria cocos fungus) eliminates dampness and improves digestion. If there is excess dampness, it will congeal into phlegm which is sticky and difficult to move.

Zi Su Ye (perilla leaf) aids digestion and helps move stuck energy in the throat, chest and abdomen.

Sheng Jiang (fresh ginger rhizome) assists the stomach and digestive energy, harmonizing digestion and helping to warm the stomach and improve the downward movement of stomach Qi. It also helps to dissolve phlegm.

Dosage: 8 pills three times per day.

BI XIE FEN QING WAN
Dioscorea Hypoglauca to Separate the Pure from the Impure Pills
Teachings of Zhu Dan-Xi
(Dou Zhen Shi Yi Xin Fu)
Dr. Zhu Dan-Xi, 1481 A.D.

Common Usage: Frequent, difficult urination; milk-like, cloudy urine.

Description: This formula is intended to eliminate urinary problems, such as thick, cloudy, milk-like urine, urinary tract infection with sometimes painful, frequent urination. The cloudy urine addressed here is often described in text books as being like "rice porridge."

Chinese Diagnosis: The small intestine, the urinary bladder and the kidney work together to separate the pure from the impure. They extract the essence from food and remove waste products from the body, recycling good Qi, clearing out the impure.

This formula strengthens the function of the kidney to remove waste, eliminate dampness (which inhibits normal functioning of the organs of elimination) and remove stagnation. When there is too much dampness in the lower part of the body, normal eliminative function is sluggish and imperfect (stagnation).

Ingredients in the Formula:
Bi Xie (dioscorea hypoglauca rhizome) separates the pure from the impure; it is important in removing damp stagnation from the lower part of the body. In Chinese Medicine, this is called cake lin. Bi Xie can be used either to resolve a case of excess damp heat, or it can strengthen kidney function.

Shi Chang Pu (acorus rhizome) opens orifices, dissolves phlegm and dampness, and assists digestion. It works to open water passages, allowing better movement of fluids in the system. This makes it easier for the body to expel dampness and stagnation.

Wu Yao (lindera root) provides the energy to improve the circulation of fluids, stops pain especially in the lower abdomen, and warms the kidney to improve the function of elimination. By improving kidney function, it helps stop frequent urination.

Yi Zhi Ren (alpinia seed) warms the kidneys, improves kidney function to stop frequent urination, and helps the kidney to better store the vital life force essence (Jing). As people age, there is a tendency to dribble urine after relieving themselves. This is caused by kidney Yang deficiency, and Yi Zhi Ren promotes kidney Yang. It also strengthens the spleen (assists digestion) which is responsible for the transformation and transportation of fluids in the body.

Fu Ling (poria cocos fungus) strengthens digestion and promotes the proper movement of water in the body. It drains excess dampness from the body and regulates the water passages.

Gan Cao (licorice root) harmonizes the other herbs and helps digestion.

Dosage: 8 pills three times per day.

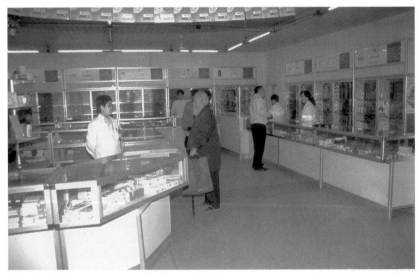

Herb shop, Beijing

BI XIE SHENG SHI WAN

Dioscorea Hypoglauca Wind Damp Formula
Subdue the Dampness Pills
The Teachings of Zhu Dan-Xi
(Dan Xi Xin Fa)
Dr. Zhu Dan-Xi, 1481 A.D.

Common Usage: Cloudy, difficult urine, chronic ulcers on the legs, ankles or feet, vaginal discharge, enlarged prostate.

Description: In Western medicine, all of the above conditions are seen as different and separate diseases, but in Chinese Medicine all are attributable to one condition: damp heat in the lower burner.

"Lower burner" is a collective term describing the combined functions of the kidney, urinary bladder, large intestine, small intestine, genitals and internal sexual organs such as the prostate, uterus and ovaries. In some books, it also includes the liver and the gall bladder. The lower burner is located below the navel. It controls the lower extremities—the legs, knees ankles and feet. Simply put, the entire triple burner—upper, middle and lower burners—control the movement of fluids in the body. All fluids which circulate below the navel must pass through the lower burner in order to get to the legs.

Chinese Diagnosis: When heat and dampness accumulate in the lower burner, the function of all areas associated with the lower burner is affected. As a consequence, urinary function is impaired, sometimes blocking it from properly draining fluids. Damp heat in the lower burner congeals the fluids which condense there, causing thick, cloudy urination, vaginal discharge and an inflamed, enlarged prostate. Additionally, it inhibits circulation of the blood and body fluids affecting the legs. This occurs because all the blood and fluids which circulate in the legs must pass through the lower burner on their way to the feet and on return.

There are three main applications of this formula: 1. Cloudy, difficult urination (chyluria); 2. White or yellow, foul smelling vaginal discharge; and 3. Chronic ulcers of the legs, ankles or feet (thromboangiitis obliterans).

Ulcers occur because the proper flow of blood and Qi are impeded as they travel to the legs which impairs healing. Thromboangiitis obliterans is a complicated condition which includes blockage or impaired movement of blood through the small and medium size arteries of the leg or foot. Early signs of impaired circulation include burning, numbness and tingling of the lower extremities.

Ingredients in the Formula:
Bi Xie Sheng Shi Wan is a variation of a classic formula called *Er Miao San* (Two Herb Marvel Powder). It contains two herbs—*Huang Bai* (phellodendron bark) and *Cang Zhu* (atractylodes lancea rhizome) which together clear damp heat from the lower burner. Cang Zhu dries dampness, strengthens the digestion to improve the processing of fluids, improves arthritic conditions of the legs, and stops vaginal discharge. Huang Bai clears heat and dampness from the lower burner and improves red, swollen and painful legs, knees, ankles and feet. It also assists the healing of urinary tract infections because of its antibiotic properties.

Bi Xie (dioscorea hypoglauca rhizome) improves kidney function (the ability to separate the pure from the impure) to eliminate dampness from the body. When kidney function is strong and healthy, fluids move properly through the lower burner, allowing the legs to move with ease.

Yi Yi Ren (coix seed) fortifies normal kidney function and improves urinary function. It contributes to this process by aiding digestion.

Mu Dan Pi (moutan peony root-bark) increases blood circulation to promote healing and helps to clear heat from the blood.

Fu Ling (poria cocos fungus) drains dampness and improves the proper movement of fluids in the body. It also aids digestion to increase assimilation of vital nutrients necessary in the healing process.

Ze Xie (alisma rhizome) improves urinary function, especially with damp heat in the lower burner. It also helps to eliminate edema.

Bai Xian Pi (dictamnus root bark) heals sores, rashes and other skin related problems by clearing heat and drying dampness.

Tong Cao (tetrapanax papyriferus pith) clears heat and drains dampness by opening water passages and promoting urination.

Zhi Zi (gardenia fruit) clears heat and dampness from all three burners, but it is especially helpful with damp heat in the lower burner. Zhi Zi clears heat from the liver channel which wraps around the genital area, assisting the treatment of vaginal discharge. It also clears heat from the blood and can help if blood appears in the urine. It also helps to relieve mental restlessness and irritability.

Note: Some of these conditions are potentially very serious. It is important to see a licensed acupuncturist who can properly diagnose and treat disease conditions. Self-medicating with this over-the-counter product is not advisable without the supervision of a licensed practitioner.

Dosage: 8 pills three times per day.

BU YANG HUAN WU WAN

Tonify Yang Qi to Restore the Other Half of the Body
Great Yang Restoration Pills
Corrections of Errors Among Physicians
(Yi Lin Gai Cuo)
Dr. Wang Qing-Ren, 1830 A.D.

Special Warning: This formula should be used only when it is certain that there is no internal bleeding and the body is maintaining a normal temperature. It should never be used when there are any types of heat signs including red face, red tongue, sweating, fever. Caution: Stroke and Paralysis are very serious conditions and self-medication is not encouraged. A patient should see a licensed practitioner, especially one who specializes in scalp acupuncture. Scalp acupuncture has proven very beneficial in China for many neurological problems, especially post-stroke paralysis.

Common Usage: Post stroke, paralysis of limbs, Bell's Palsy and Trigeminal Neuralgia.

Description: After stroke: For partial paralysis of the arms and legs, facial paralysis, slurred speech and atrophy of muscles, especially following a cerebral vascular accident (CVA). A stroke can be caused by three different conditions. The first is a passage of plaque material (made up primarily of cholesterol) which blocks narrow arteries of the brain, cutting off the blood supply to a portion of the brain. The second is an aneurysm or ballooning of a weakened blood vessel which may break, causing internal bleeding in the brain. The third is a spasm of the vessel wall causing a restriction of the flow of blood in the brain. Any of these conditions can lead to severe loss of body function.

Chinese Diagnosis: A stroke is caused by the unruly movement of internal pathogenic wind which appears as any unnatural movement in the body. When one experiences a cerebral vascular accident (wind-stroke), paralysis often impedes the normal function of one side of the body. Dr. Wang felt that individuals lost the use of one half of their yang Qi as the result of a CVA. Usually a stroke blocks the free flow of Yang Qi on one side of the body, allowing for blood and Qi in the meridians to congeal and stagnate. It can be said that this formula opens up the meridians which have become constricted because of a stroke and helps promote free flow of Qi and blood to paralyzed areas.

If the meridians are blocked, the yang Qi that animates the body cannot flow freely to areas of atrophy. The goal of this formula is to open the channels (meridians) so that Qi once again flows freely. Qi moves blood, and if the Qi flows freely, the blood will follow. If the blood produces enough Qi, the Qi will help move the blood and healing nutrients can flow to areas which need to heal.

Ingredients in the Formula:

Huang Qi (astragalus root) directs Qi, opening the meridians. It also directs Qi toward the head and to the outer parts of the body where healing needs to occur.

Di Long (lumbricus; dried earthworm) opens the meridians and stops muscle spasms and numbness. It is used to unblock stagnation and to promote the movement of stiff, painful joints, to improve range of motion and to eliminate hemiplegia (paralysis of one side of the body).

Hong Hua (safflower) and *Tao Ren* (peach kernel) are paired herbs that invigorate blood, help break up stagnant blood and open up blockage in the blood vessels.

Chi Shao (red peony root) moves blood and breaks up stagnation. It works along with Dang Gui (angelica sinensis root) to direct blood to areas of resistance.

Chuan Xiong (ligusticum root) breaks up stagnation of Qi and blood. Chuan Xiong also expels pathogenic wind and directs the energy of the herbs to the head where the damage originally occurred. It stops headache pain, dizziness and numbness.

Dosage: 8 pills three times per day.

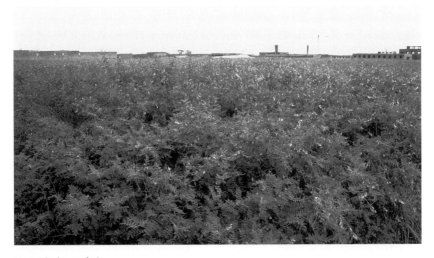

Huang Qi (astragalus)

CHAI HU LONG GU MU LI WAN

Bupleurum Dragon Bone Oyster Shell Pills
Discussion of Cold-Induced Disorders
(Shang Han Lun)
Dr. Chang Chung-Ching, 142–220 A.D.

Common Usage: Irregular heartbeat, calms emotions.

Description: This formula regulates the heartbeat, stops palpitations, calms the emotions and alleviates irritability. It can help those who have been frightened and continue to be affected by that fright.

Chinese Diagnosis: This formula was originally intended to treat what is called the Three Yang Stages of disease. A patient gets a common cold which simultaneously attacks three levels of the body. It addresses Tai Yang stage (a more superficial common cold), Shao Yang stage (halfway between the superficial and deeper layers; see discussion of Xiao Chai Hu Tang Wan) and Yang Ming Level, (a deeper layer) which is characterized by the "four bigs": big sweating, big thirst, big fever and big pulse.

In more modern times, this formula has come to be used more for such conditions as irritability and palpitations. It calms anger and settles the heartbeat, especially a heartbeat that becomes irregular with exercise.

Symptoms include anger, irritability, palpitations, and most importantly, a bloated, tight chest accompanied by a feeling of fullness in the chest.

Ingredients in the Formula:

Xiao Chai Hu Tang Wan (Minor Bupleurum; see page 114) harmonizes the body, calms the liver and gallbladder and eliminates phlegm.

Da Huang (rhubarb root) clears intense internal heat, calms the emotions and purges constipation.

Gui Zhi (cinnamon twig) regulates the heartbeat, encourages blood flow and breaks up stagnation which may be blocking normal body function.

Long Gu (dragon bone) and *Mu Li* (oyster shell) calm the spirit and settle the emotions by sinking the restless yang energy which wants to flood upward in the body to disturb the mind. In Chinese Medicine, the heart controls the mind and emotions, together described as spirit. Long Gu and Mu Li pull down excess yang energy and sink it into the body where it belongs and where it will not disturb the heart or the mind.

Fu Ling (poria cocos fungus) drains dampness, regulates digestion and ensures proper distribution of fluids throughout the body. It also assists in calming the restless mind.

Dosage: 8 pills three times per day.

CHAI HU SHU GAN WAN

Bupleurum Soothe Liver Pills
Collected Treatises of Zhang Jing-Yue
(Jing Yue Quan Shu)
Dr. Zhang Jing-Yue, 1624 A.D.

Common Usage: Relieves stress, warms hands and feet, regulates the menses.

Description: Frigid hands and feet are often caused by constricted emotions which entrap yang heat within the body, preventing it from flowing smoothly to the extremities where it can warm the skin and muscles. This condition is frequently found in women and is created by blockage of emotions. This type of stagnation can also cause irregular or abnormal menstruation, especially with accompanying cramps and pain often brought on by stress.

It can sometimes appear as false cold in which the patient is not ill, but can be experiencing discomfort. Symptoms may include abdominal or chest pain, alternating constipation and diarrhea, difficult or painful menses, as well as cold hands and feet.

Based on Si Ni San (Frigid Extremities Powder), from the *Shang Han Lun (Discussion of Cold-Induced Disorders)*, written by Dr. Chang Chung-Ching (142–220 A.D.), Chai Hu Shu Gan Wan warms hands and feet, alleviates stress and helps to harmonize the emotions.

Ingredients in the Formula:
Chai Hu (bupleurum root) regulates the liver, assists in harmonizing the spleen and stomach, and relieves liver Qi Stagnation. When the liver is soft and relaxed, the body's flow of energy is released and the heat from within can circulate to the hands and feet.

Bai Shao (white peony root) clears heat, regulates and nourishes liver blood and protects the body from the loss of too much essential fluid.

Zhi Ke (aurantium fruit) breaks up stagnation in the middle of the body and directs it downward.

Gan Cao (licorice root) harmonizes the functions of the other herbs.

Chuan Xiong (ligusticum root) invigorates Qi and blood to improve circulation. It also normalizes the menstrual cycle and can help alleviate pain due to difficult menstruation.

Xiang Fu (cyperus rhizome) alleviates constricted liver Qi, helps to harmonize the digestive functions of the body, and helps to normalize the menstrual cycle.

Dosage: 8 pills three times a day.

DA CHAI HU WAN

Major Bupleurum Pills
Discussion of Cold-Induced Disorders
(Shang Han Lun)
Dr. Chang Chung-Ching, 142–220 A.D.

Common Usage: Common cold moving internally with heat signs.

Description: A variation of Xiao Chai Hu Tang Wan (Minor Bupleurum; see page 114), Da Chai Hu Wan treats a severe case of Shao Yang Syndrome and Yang Ming heat together. It harmonizes and clears severe heat.

Chinese Diagnosis: When an individual gets sick and is unable to fight off the common cold, it can move inward to a deeper level of the body where there is a fight between the body's immune system and the illness. In this case, the illness has invaded a deeper layer of the body and is causing major discomfort.

Symptoms include intermittent chills and fever, painful, bloated chest, nausea, firm stomach or abdomen, constipation, or possible diarrhea.

Ingredients in the Formula:
Ban Xia (pinellia rhizome), *Chai Hu* (bupleurum root), *Gan Jiang* (dry ginger rhizome), *Huang Qin* (scutellaria root), *Da Zao* (black jujube date) harmonize digestion, clear excess heat, and fight the illness. Both Chai Hu and Huang Qin have antibiotic properties. Chai Hu in particular reduces a fever, stops cough, and is both anti-bacterial and antiviral. Huang Qin can reduce a fever and has antibiotic properties.

Da Huang (rhubarb root) clears intense excess internal heat and purges constipation, purging heat through the stool. It also has antibiotic properties which inhibits the growth of various bacteria.

Zhi Shi (aurantium fruit) breaks up Qi stagnation and clears Yang Ming heat from the intestines.

Bai Shao (white peony root) clears heat, stops pain and spasms. It also helps to harmonize the Qi which fights infections both internally and on the surface of the body.

Dosage: 8 pills three times per day.

DA HUANG JIANG ZHI WAN

Rhubarb Reduce Fat Pills
Rhubarb Tea Pills
Modern Concentrated Formula

Note: It is not a good idea to rely on laxatives as a weight-loss solution. This is intended for short-term intestinal fullness. Do not use often.

Common Usage: Purgative, very strong laxative.

Description: For someone with very strongly impacted stool or who is simply unable to move the bowels with gentler laxatives. It is intended here as a short-term means of weight loss. Laxatives can reduce fat by clearing bowels that are slow to move and purging food when one overeats.

It can be taken when someone has a high fever with profuse sweating, a strong thirst, constipation, abdominal fullness and pain. The idea here is to purge the heat along with the accumulated, sometimes impacted stool. When there is a bowel movement, the internal heat of the body is reduced.

Ingredients in the Formula:
Da Huang (rhubarb root and rhizome) is a strong laxative.

Dosage: 3 pills three times per day.

DAN SHEN YIN WAN

Red Sage Drink Pills
Salvia Tea Pills
Collected Songs about Contemporary Formulas
(Shi Fang Ge Kuo)
Chen Nian-Zi, 1801 A.D.

Special Warning: Angina pain may be a warning sign for a very serious health condition. It sometimes occurs before a heart attack. Please see a licensed health care practitioner immediately.

Common Usage: Chest pain, angina, stomach pain.

Description: This three-herb formula is used to stop chest or stomach pain. It assists the body when there is stagnation of blood or Qi in the chest and stomach. Pain may be present, and these herbs break up stagnation which is causing that pain.

Chinese Diagnosis: Any time Qi is blocked, there can also be a stagnation of blood. This formula breaks up stagnant Qi and stagnant blood so both flow freely through the chest and stomach area. This prescription can be used for any of the following conditions: Peptic ulcers, chronic pancreatitis, chronic gastritis, chronic hepatitis, cholecystitis (gallbladder pain and congestion), and angina.

Ingredients in the Formula:
Dan Shen (salvia root) is the main herb given to patients in China who are having heart problems. It invigorates blood so that it doesn't stagnate. It helps open blood vessels, especially coronary arteries, so that blood can move smoothly through the heart and the entire circulatory system. It reduces chest pain and calms the spirit.

Tan Xiang (sandalwood) breaks up blockage in the chest, reduces pain and has been used recently in China to treat coronary artery disease.

Sha Ren (amomum fruit) improves digestion and eliminates dampness. In the terminology of Chinese Medicine, cholesterol in the bloodstream and the build-up of deposits on artery walls are known as dampness and phlegm. Sha Ren prevents dampness and the stagnation that dampness creates.

Note: In Chinese hospitals, heart patients are often given a Dan Shen liquid extract IV for treatment of heart disease and to stop heart attacks. Dan Shen opens up the coronary arteries and improves blood flow to nourish the heart muscle and to improve heart function.

Dosage: 8 pills three times per day.

DING CHUAN WAN

Stop Asthma Pills
Clear Mountain Air Tea Pills
Exquisite Formulas for Fostering Longevity
(Fu Shou Jing Fan)
Dr. Wu Min, 1530 A.D.

Common Usage: Stops wheezing (asthma), cough, and chronic bronchitis.

Description: This prescription was designed to treat chronic asthma and to stop wheezing. It assists in reducing the intensity of an acute asthma attack with thick, copious, yellow or white, sticky phlegm. It can be taken to help clear heat in the lungs and ease the constriction of phlegm in the bronchials. It helps to open air passages and to utilize oxygen more efficiently. It will help to stop associated coughing from thick, copious phlegm.

It can also be taken for chronic or acute bronchitis when there is phlegm which inhibits breathing.

Ingredients in the Formula:

Bai Guo (ginkgo biloba nut) stops wheezing and expels excess phlegm. It also strengthens the lungs and improves breathing.

Sang Bai Pi (mulberry root bark) stops wheezing, coughing and clears heat from the lungs.

Bai Bu (stemona root) stops both acute and chronic coughing.

Xing Ren (apricot seed) and *Zi Su Zi* (perilla seed) stop coughing and wheezing and help the body to utilize oxygen more efficiently. This concept in Chinese Medicine is called "grasping the Qi." It refers to the idea that there is Qi in the air which the lungs extract when we breathe. It is said that Qi is "grasped" by the kidneys. The kidneys control the bones and bone marrow where blood is produced. When the kidneys are strong, the body produces healthy blood with plenty of red blood cells which collect oxygen from the alveoli in the lungs.

When Lung Qi is rebellious, the energy goes upward in the throat, causing a cough. Xing Ren and Zi Su Zi direct Lung Qi downward in its normal direction.

Zi Wan (aster root) stops many types of cough and expels phlegm.

Huang Qin (scutellaria root) clears heat from the lungs, expels thick, sticky yellow phlegm and functions as a natural antibiotic to fight infections in the chest.

Jie Geng (platycodon root) stops cough, expels phlegm and strengthens the lungs. It directs the energy of the other herbs in this formula to the lungs where they can be more effective.

Ban Xia (pinellia rhizome) is the main herb in Chinese Medicine to clear phlegm from the lungs. It also directs rebellious Qi downward. People with asthma often feel that they can't take a breath because their lungs are already full. This feeling is sometimes caused by rebellious Lung Qi which will not descend and leaves the lungs feeling full. Ban Xia and other herbs in this formula have the property of directing Lung Qi downward where it can be "grasped" and utilized by the body.

Gan Cao (licorice root) harmonizes the formula, supports the lungs, and the digestion.

Dosage: 8 pills three times per day.

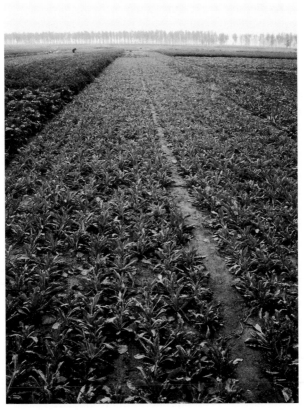

Da Qing Ye (isatis leaf)

DU HUO JI SHENG WAN

Angelica Pubescens and Sang Ji Sheng Pills
Solitary Hermit
Thousand Ducat Formulas
(Qian Jin Yao Fang)
Dr. Sun Si-Miao, 652 A.D.

Common Usage: Lower back pain, sciatica, arthritis.

Description: Especially beneficial for the elderly or weak, Du Huo Ji Sheng Wan treats many types of body pain including lower back pain, sciatica, ruptured discs, and knee problems. It also helps alleviate rheumatic arthritis, bone disorders, chronic osteoarthritis and any type of condition that affects the bones and muscles. It focuses primarily on the lower back and knees.

As people age, muscle and joint pain becomes more prevalent. This formula contains many nourishing herbs which fortify the body and alleviate pain which occurs primarily as the body degenerates. Chinese Medicine says that as we age, kidney energy decreases. Since kidneys control the lower part of the body, this formula contains herbs that strengthen the kidneys.

Ingredients in the Formula:

Many of the herbs in this formula are found in *Ba Zhen Wan* (see page 55) which contains two herb formulas (Four Gentlemen and Four Substances). One improves digestion and the assimilation of nutrients; the other nourishes blood. When there is enough Qi and blood and both are circulating freely in the body, there is no pain.

Ren Shen (panax ginseng root), *Fu Ling* (poria cocos fungus), *Gan Cao* (licorice root), *Sheng Di Huang* (raw rhemannia root), Dang Gui (angelica sinensis root), *Chuan Xiong* (ligusticum root) improve digestion, build blood, and regulate both Qi and blood.

Du Zhong (eucommia bark) strengthens the kidneys and the lower back, nourishes the tendons and bones, and helps promote circulation of Qi and blood.

Du Huo (angelica pubescens root) is the main herb to help the lower back and to stop back pain, both in acute and chronic cases. It helps relieve the discomfort of arthritis, especially in the lower back, by expelling wind and drying dampness.

Sang Ji Sheng (mulberry parasite) nourishes the liver and the kidneys, strengthens the lower back and knees, and helps to build blood and body fluids. Strong blood and fluids balance the drying and warming properties of the other herbs in this formula.

Rou Gui (cinnamon bark) warms the kidneys and helps build vitality. It is said in Chinese Medicine that as people age, their vitality wanes and often the fire of life grows cold. Rou Gui stokes digestive fire and warms the interior which leads to a warming of all channels of the body.

Qin Jiao (gentiana macrophylla root), *Fang Feng* (siler; ledebouriella root), *Niu Xi* (acyranthes root), and *Xi Xin* (asarium herb; wild ginger) improve circulation, soften tendons, and assist the other herbs in the elimination of arthritis symptoms.

Dosage: 8 pills three times per day.

FANG FENG TONG SHENG WAN

Siler to Release the Exterior Pills
Ledebouriella Sagely Unblocks
Formulas from the Discussion Illuminating
the Yellow Emperor's Basic Questions
(Huang di Su Wen Xuan Ming Lun Fang)
Dr. Liu Yuan-Su, 1172 A.D.

Common Usage: Common cold becoming worse.

Description: This is a complicated formula intended to be taken when a common cold doesn't improve. It is said in Chinese Medicine that a common cold attacks the body in the most superficial meridians—the skin layer. The treatment of choice in the initial stages is to induce a sweat.

In this situation, either the sweating treatment did not work or the body is not strong enough to resist the illness. The illness remains lodged in the superficial layers of the body and is now starting to move deeper.

Fang Feng Tong Sheng Wan combines two methods of treatment—fighting an infection with antibiotic herbs and nourishing and strengthening the body to resist the deeper invasion of illness.

Symptoms include aversion to cold, chills and fever, dizziness, bitter taste in the mouth, dry mouth, red, sore eyes, sore throat, tight chest, constipation, urinary difficulty with possible bloody urine, and nasal congestion.

Ingredients in the Formula:

Lian Qiao (forsythia fruit) reduces fever and fights infection.

Huang Qin (scutellaria root) clears heat from the chest, throat, lungs and chest as well as fights infection.

Jing Jie (schizonepeta herb) fights the two most common types of colds—wind-heat and wind-cold. It helps produce sweating to clear heat.

Fang Feng (siler; ledebouriella root) guards against wind and causes the pores of the skin to open and the body to sweat.

Zhi Zi (gardenia fruit) clears heat from all areas of the body and helps to alleviate irritability associated with fever.

Bai Shao (white peony root) guards against excessive sweating, stops muscle spasms, and builds resistance by nourishing blood.

Da Huang (rhubarb root) clears heat from the body by purging the bowels. It also has antibiotic properties.

Bo He (mint herb) reduces a fever, encourages sweating and clears heat and inflammation from the face and eyes, improving a sore throat.

Chuang Xiong (ligusticum root) increases blood flow to the brain to help alleviate a headache.

Jie Geng (platycodon root) strengthens the lungs, clears heat and infection from the lungs, stops sore throat and helps to improve immunity by assisting digestion and allowing the body to disperse protective Qi (Wei Qi) throughout the body.

Bai Zhu (atractylodes rhizome) improves digestion and works with the other herbs to protect the surface layer of the body from external invasion by pathogens.

Dang Gui (angelica sinensis root) nourishes blood and strengthens the constitution so that the body can better resist illness.

Gan Cao (licorice root) harmonizes the diverse elements of this formula which is very complicated and includes herbs to fight infection, strengthen the body and to improve digestion.

Gan Jiang (dried ginger rhizome) improves digestion, stops nausea and helps to induce sweating to expel the foreign evil.

Dosage: 8 pills three times per day.

FANG JI HUANG QI WAN

Stephania and Astragalus Pills
Essentials from the Golden Cabinet
(Jin Gui Yao Lue)
Dr. Chang Chung-Ching, 142–220 A.D.

Common Usage: Arthritis, rheumatoid arthritis.

Description: This formula treats two kinds of conditions: A sudden attack of superficial skin edema anywhere on the body, or a swollen, damp type of arthritis. Both conditions are associated with dampness and urinary bladder difficulties. Body fluids suddenly start collecting under the skin and cause discomfort and movement problems.

Chinese Diagnosis: It is said that there is an underlying deficiency of Wei Qi, the Qi that protects the exterior of the body from external invasion by pathogens. In this case, the deficiency allows dampness to invade the body and cause discomfort. Treatment begins with strengthening the Wei Qi and draining dampness, opening the pores of the skin to force out dampness through sweat.

Symptoms include sweating, chills, difficult or scanty urination, edema anywhere on the body, sometimes palpitations of the heart, numbness, swelling or stiffness. It can be associated with rheumatic heart disease, nephritis, and arthritis—numb, swollen, puffy with difficulty in moving joints.

Ingredients in the Formula:

Han Fang Ji (stephania tetrandra root) acts as a diuretic, draining fluids through the bladder. In so doing, it helps alleviate the pain and discomfort of muscles and joints.

Huang Qi (astragalus root) strengthens Wei Qi, stabilizes the exterior of the body and promotes the immune system to ward off disease.

Bai Zhu (atractylodes rhizome) aids digestion, dries dampness and helps to promote Wei Qi (defensive Qi).

Gan Jiang (dried ginger rhizome) harmonizes the digestion and warms the stomach to combat dampness and cold. Improving digestion helps elevate levels of leukocytes or white blood cells which fight infections and disease.

Gan Cao (licorice root) and *Da Zao* (black jujube dates) harmonize the formula and aid digestion.

Dosage: 8 pills three times per day.

GAN MAI DA ZAO WAN

Licorice, Wheat and Jujube Date Pills
Calm Spirit Tea Pills
Settle Shen
Essentials of the Golden Cabinet
(Jin Gui Yao Lue)
Dr. Chang Chung-Ching, 142–220 A.D.

Common Usage: Menopause, mood swings, anxiety, depression.

Description: Gan Mai Da Zao Wan is a classic formula of three herbs, a treatment for a menopausal woman's condition called "dry organ syndrome." It is intended for yin-deficient, pre-menopausal or menopausal women whose internal organs are not being properly nourished by blood and body fluids. This occurs as women age and their kidney energy decreases so that internal organs are affected by internal heat and dryness.

Chinese Diagnosis: In particular, this condition affects the heart, liver and spleen (digestive system). If the digestive system weakens, it doesn't produce enough blood or transport body fluids to the proper locations. The liver stores the blood and it doesn't work effectively if there is not enough blood volume. Without enough liver blood, the heart isn't properly nourished. In Chinese Medicine, the heart is the most important organ in controlling anxiety. The heart works along with the liver to maintain a healthy emotional equilibrium.

Symptoms include flushed face, hot flashes, mood swings, melancholy and unaccountable crying, restless sleep with night sweats, and odd behavior. So called "odd behavior," such as excessive worry, anxiety and unexplained fears, is usually considered psychosomatic by Western Medicine and would be treated with anti-depressants which often aggravate the underlying condition of dryness.

Ingredients in the Formula:
The three herbs that make up the original formula are *Gan Cao* (licorice root), *Fu Xiao Mai* (triticum aestivium seed) and *Da Zao* (black jujube dates). The original formula was intended as a food treatment, to be taken long term for best results. In pill form, the formula has been expanded to include four more herbs.

Fu Xiao Mai (triticum aestivium seed) stops sweating, nourishes the heart, calms the spirit, and reduces insomnia, emotional instability and anxiety.

Gan Cao (licorice root) moistens the stomach and digestive organs as it harmonizes the herbs in this formula.

Da Zao (black jujube dates) moistens dryness in the stomach and digestive tract and tonifies Qi.

Fu Ling (Poria cocos fungus) aids digestion, helps normalize the functioning of fluids in the body, and moistens dry organs.

He Shou Wu (polygonum multiflorium root) builds blood. By making more blood, especially liver blood which nourishes the heart, He Shou Wu assists all the organs to relieve stress, anxiety, insomnia and emotional upset.

Bai He (lily bulb) opens the channels of the heart and eliminates stagnation in the chest.

He Huan Pi (albizzia bark) is called the "happy herb." It elevates the spirit, combats depression, insomnia and irritability.

Note: This formula is intended to be taken long term because it moistens and nourishes the body without any negative side effects. Because the condition that it treats is long-standing and has taken many years to evolve, it is going to take this formula some time to begin to alleviate the symptoms. The main ingredients in this formula are sold in almost every Chinese market world wide. They can be made into tea and consumed every day by women who have the above symptoms or who want to prevent their occurrence. See Appendix in the back of the book for bulk Chinese herb companies.

Dosage: 8 pills three times per day.

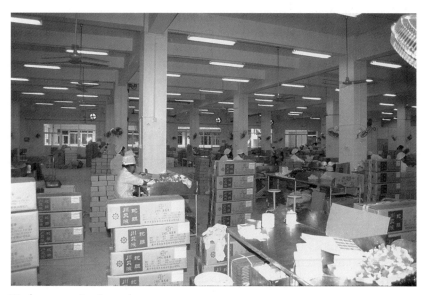

Warehouse processing, Pangaoshou

GE GEN WAN

Kudzu Formula Pills
Kudzu Tea Pills
Discussion of Cold-Induced Disorders
(Shang Han Lun)
Dr. Chang Chung-Ching, 142–220 A.D.

Common Usage: Common cold with neck pain.

Description: There are several different types of common colds and many variations of formulas to treat them. The type of treatment depends on the symptoms which are, in this case, wind-cold with a stiff neck. It is very common with some types of common colds to get achy muscles and a stiff neck. The Chinese say that wind invades the body at the base of the neck, and it is this location that is most vulnerable with certain types of cold conditions.

Chinese Diagnosis: Wind-cold symptoms include chills, maybe a slight fever without sweating, a headache, bodyaches, upper back pain, a stiff neck and a stuffy nose with clear or white mucus.

The intent of this formula is to cause sweating that forces the pathogenic bacteria or virus out of the body.

Ingredients in the Formula:
Chai Hu (bupleurum root), *Huang Qin* (scutellaria root), *Qiang Huo* (notopterygium root), *Bai Zhi* (angelica dahurica root) have antibiotic properties, reduce a fever, and fight acute infectious diseases.

Shi Gao (gypsum) strongly clears heat to reduce a fever.

Sheng Jiang (fresh ginger rhizome) is a diaphoretic (causes sweating) and helps relieve infections in the upper respiratory tract. It also helps to break of phlegm stagnation and to improve breathing.

Gui Zhi (cinnamon twig) opens the pores and causes the body to sweat in order to reduce a fever.

Bai Shao (white peony root) prevents the body from sweating too much. Bai Shao combined with Gan Cao is a two-herb formula, *Shao Yao Gan Cao Tang* (Peony and Licorice Formula), for eliminating muscle spasms, neck stiffness, aches and pain.

Gan Cao (licorice root), *Da Zao* (black jujube dates) and *Gan Jiang* (dried ginger rhizome) harmonize digestion and help to strengthen the body by improving the assimilation of nutrients and by harmonizing the interior and exterior of the body.

Ma Huang (ephedra herb) works with Gui Zhi to open the pores and reduce a fever through perspiration. This formula relies on one of the basic treatment methods of Chinese Medicine, the sweating method, and Ma Huang is a diaphoretic (an herb that causes sweating). Ma Huang also opens the lungs and bronchials so that an individual can breathe more easily, eliminating wheezing and the obstruction of breathing passages.

Ge Gen (pueraria; kudzu root) releases a stiff neck and reduces neck pain.

Dosage: 8 pills three times per day.

GUAN JIE YAN WAN
Joint Inflammation Pills
Clear Damp Heat Channel Blockage
Modern Formula

Warning: Anyone with red, inflamed joints should not use this product. Many herbs in this formula have warming properties which would possibly aggravate a condition in which heat signs are present. It is best to use this product under the guidance of a trained acupuncturist.

Common Usage: Arthritis, rheumatism, sciatica, aching joints.

Description: This prescription is for those with either chronic or acute joint pain, including low back pain, cold, achy knees or ankles, or swollen, puffy knees or ankles. It reduces swelling and helps to eliminate pain. It can also be used by those with stiff shoulders and painful elbows and wrists.

Ingredients in the Formula:
Cang Zhu (atractylodes lancea rhizome) eliminates swelling and dampness and stops arthritis pain.

Yi Yi Ren (coix seed) eliminates dampness and swelling, increases joint flexibility and stops muscle spasms.

Zhe Tong Pi (zanthoxylum ailanthoides bark) improves lower back pain, knee pain and eliminates spasms in the arms and legs.

Huang Qin (scutellaria root) clears heat and inflammation.

Han Fang Ji (stephania tetrandra root) opens channels, clears heat and relieves red, hot, swollen, painful inflammation. Many other herbs in this formula have warming properties which possibly may make red, inflamed joints worse.

Qin Jiao (gentiana macrophylla root) stops cramping and pain, relaxes muscles and tendons, especially in the arms and legs.

Chuan Niu Xi (achyranthes root) strengthens joints, tendons and bones, and it is beneficial in improving mobility in stiff joints, especially for the lower back and knees.

Gui Zhi (cinnamon twig) improves circulation, warms the channels, driving out cold that causes pain, and helps move the blood while breaking up stagnation and dampness. Gui Zhi has the property of directing the warming effects of the formula to the hands and feet, thus being helpful for those who have stiff fingers and toes.

Du Huo (angelica pubescens root) improves stiffness and pain of the lower back, knees and legs.

Jiang Huang (curcuma longa rhizome) reduces pain and inflammation in the upper back and shoulders.

Ma Huang (ephedra herb) helps by relieving dampness near the surface of the skin, reducing inflammation and pain.

Chuan Wu (aconitum carmichaeli root) and *Cao Wu* (aconitum kusnezoffi root) eliminate cold and stop pain, and are therefore very valuable in treating arthritis conditions in older people.

Gan Jiang (dry ginger rhizome) warms digestion and helps to eliminate pain.

Dosage: 8 pills three times per day.

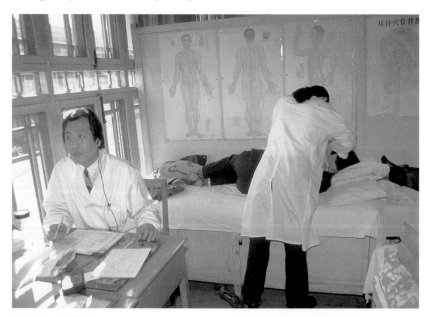

TCM Hospital, Beijing

HAI MA BU SHEN WAN

Sea Horse Tonic Pills
The English-Chinese Encyclopedia of Practical
Traditional Chinese Medicine, Vol. #5
Chief Editor Xu Xiang-Cai, 1989 A.D.

Warning: This product is warm and should not be taken by anyone who shows any type of heat signs.

Common Usage: General tonic, impotence, reduced sex drive.

Description: This formula is designed for those who are weak and in need of fortification. It can be used by older people who experience fatigue, impotence, low back pain, cold hands and feet. The formula will also benefit women following childbirth when their Qi and blood are exhausted. It can also be taken by those recovering from a extended illness and in need of rebuilding their strength and energy.

Chinese Diagnosis: The kidneys are the foundation of good health. As someone gets older, the kidney Qi naturally begins to wane. This formula specifically works to rebuild kidney strength. It also improves digestion, improves blood circulation, thus improving overall health.

Ingredients in the Formula:

Shu Di Huang (prepared rehmannia root) and *Dang Gui* (angelica sinensis root) nourish blood. Shu Di Huang also nourishes Yin fluids and Jing (vital life force essence). It is said that as people age, their bodies and vital essence dry out. Fluids, which nourish organs and lubricate muscles and bones, are restored by this formula. Dang Gui also helps to eliminate arthritis pain by invigorating blood to improve circulation.

Fu Zi (prepared aconite root) warms the fire of life. As people age, their life force energy diminishes; the fire of life wanes within them. Fu Zi promotes the function of the heart (fire), improves circulation and warms the muscles and tendons to stop arthritis pain. It lifts yang energy and counteracts impotence.

Yin Yang Huo (epimedium leaf), *Bu Gu Zhi* (psoralea fruit) and *Tu Si Zi* (cuscuta seed) strengthen kidney function, especially kidney Yang which controls sexual energy in both men and women. Yin Yang Huo eliminates low back pain and impotence as it dispels the pain of arthritis. Bu Gu Zhi restores Jing (vital sexual essence), aids digestion (which restores the health of the whole body) and stops pain in the lower back and knees. Tu Si Zi nourishes both kidney Yin and Yang, as well as kidney Jing (vital essence). It also improves vision, ear ringing and blurry vision.

Ren Shen (panax ginseng root) and *Dang Shen* (codonopsis root) improve digestion and elevate energy levels. Ren Shen is especially popular as a tonic for older men to restore sexual function, but it is even more valuable in replenishing Yuan Qi (source Qi). Both Ren Shen and Dang Shen strengthen lung function, assist digestion and build energy. Dang Shen is often used as a less expensive substitute for the much more expensive Ren Shen.

Lu Shen (donkey kidney) and *Lu Gen* (deer tendons) restore animal strength. In Chinese Medicine, a concept has evolved from the shamanic tradition that theorizes that to be as strong as an animal, you need to eat animal bones and animal flesh. While the root of this idea appears during prehistory, modern research has shown that many of these substances have properties imagined thousands of years ago. Donkey kidney makes the kidney function much stronger. Eating deer tendons strengthens human tendons.

Fu Pen Zi (rubus fruit) warms the kidney, restores the life force essence and restrains the essence so that the body will retain it.

Niu Xi (achyranthes root) strengthens tendons and bones, supports liver and kidneys, and breaks up stagnation. It improves joint mobility, nourishes the muscles and stops arthritis pain.

Wu Yao (lindera root) warms kidney fire, regulates Qi and breaks up cold stagnation throughout the body.

Dosage: 8 pills three times per day.

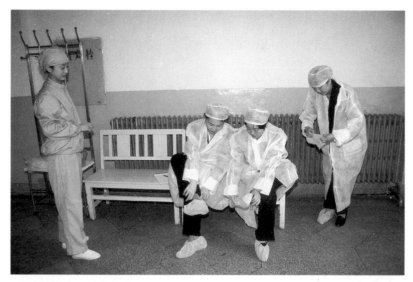

Dressing in sterile clothing before a factory inspection

HAI ZAO WAN

Sargassum Seaweed Pills
Modern Formula

A single herb formula, Hai Zao is used to promote normal thyroid function. The iodine in Hai Zao regulates and normalizes the function of the thyroid, for those who have metabolism problems or other difficulties including minor goiter, swelling of the thyroid gland on the neck. Hai Zao also helps to reduce swelling and nodules on the neck.

Dosage: 8 pills three times per day.

HUAN SHAO DAN

Restore Youth Pills
Return to Youth
Support Jing, Earth, and Water
Treatise on Prescriptions
Dr. Ren Zhai, Date Unknown

Note: This formula should be taken only by someone with a very weak pulse and a pale tongue. Anyone with a red tongue and any signs of internal heat should not use this formula. Women tend toward yin deficiency and often experience hot flashes or sensations of heat on the face and neck. Women with these symptoms should not take this formula because it will aggravate heat conditions.

Common Usage: Impotence, old age, fatigue.

Description: This formula is designed to replenish youthful energy. It can be used by either men or women to assist in replenishing sexual energy and vigor.

Chinese Diagnosis: Restores kidney Yang. As people age, their kidney energy begins to diminish. Kidney energy contains Jing (the life force essence) which is lost in the aging process and through various lifestyle abuses. Such abuses include excessive sex, alcohol and drug abuse, as well as eating a poor diet. People also age because of an over-reliance on stimulants such as coffee, cigarettes and junk food.

Symptoms of aging include impotence, frequent urination at night, lower back pain, knee pain or sore knees, dizziness, amnesia, Alzheimer's disease, short-term memory loss (forgetfulness), poor appetite and a very weak pulse.

Ingredients in the Formula:

Shu Di Huang (prepared rehmannia root) nourishes blood and Yin (essential body fluids), as well as Jing (the life force essence). It can help alleviate old age symptoms such as gray hair, lower back pain, impotence, ear ringing, hearing loss and mental forgetfulness. It also strengthens kidney function which controls the lower parts of the body—ankles, knees and lower back.

Gou Qi Zi (lycium fruit) strengthens both liver and kidneys, nourishes both yin and blood, and replenishes the life force essence. It is especially valuable for treating eye problems such as blurry vision and loss of vision.

Bi Xie (dioscorea hypoglauca rhizome) improves kidney function, thereby improving urinary function and the ability of the kidney to separate the pure from the impure. It is used for cloudy, milky urine, and other types of urinary difficulty.

Fu Ling (poria cocos fungus) strengthens digestion and transports fluids to their proper place in the body. Its main function in this formula is to drain excess dampness and to clear phlegm stagnation.

Ba Ji Tian (morinda root) and *Rou Cong Rong* (cistanches stem) strengthen the kidney yang (the fire of life), warming cold hands and feet, improving urinary function, and strengthening the lower back and knees. Rou Cong Rong can also eliminate constipation, a common problem in older people.

Xiao Hui Xiang (fennel seed) warms the interior of the body, expels cold and harmonizes the stomach. It helps alleviate indigestion and is often served in Middle Eastern nations and in India following a meal to enhance digestion.

Du Zhong (eucommia bark) enhances the function of the liver and kidneys, strengthens the tendons and bones, and improves circulation of Qi and blood. It has also been used recently to lower high blood pressure.

Niu Xi (achyranthes root) assists the normal functions of tendons and bones, lower back and knees. It improves liver and kidneys and can help dizziness, headache and mental clarity. It also has been shown to lower blood pressure and to stop pain caused by arthritis.

Wu Wei Zi (schisandra fruit) improves breathing by strengthening normal lung function. It stops coughs and calms the spirit. It works as a natural tranquilizer to calm and quiet someone who is restless and agitated. It also strengthens the kidneys, improving the function of the bladder.

Da Zao (black jujube dates) harmonizes the middle—stomach and digestive organs—and elevates Qi to improve overall body energy.

Shan Zhu Yu (cornus fruit) strengthens the kidneys and helps to contain Jing (the life force essence). It nourishes both the liver and the kidneys, helping the low back and knees. It also alleviates lightheadedness and dizziness, improving mental clarity.

Zhu Shi Zi (papyrifera fruit) tonifies kidney function, improves vision, and supports the loins and genitals.

Dosage: 8 pills three times per day.

HUANG LIAN JIE DU WAN
Coptis Clear Toxins Pills
Arcane Essentials from the Imperial Library
(Wai Tai Bi Yao)
Dr. Wang Tao, 752 A.D.

Warning: Anyone who is seriously ill should see a licensed practitioner and should not attempt home treatment. If someone you know exhibits strong fever, dry mouth and throat, incoherence, insomnia, vomits blood, or passes bloody diarrhea, send them to a hospital.

Common Usage: Natural antibiotic, skin infections, dysentery, sore throat, ear infections.

Description: This formula was originally prescribed for patients with a serious infection, exhibiting such signs as a strong fever, irritability, dry mouth and dry throat. Other associated symptoms included incoherence and insomnia accompanied by some type of skin lesion, carbuncle, boil or other skin infection with pus.

Today, such conditions are usually treated in a hospital, thus limiting this formula's modern usage to treating conditions like skin eruptions, dysentery, sore throat, ear infections, or urinary tract infections requiring a natural antibiotic.

Huang Lian Jie Du Wan can be used for jaundice, septicemia (systemic infection), and pneumonia (please see warning above).

Chinese Diagnosis: Such a condition is called heat and toxins. Any time there is infection with inflammation, red inflamed sores, swollen lymph glands, an infected wound with redness affecting the surrounding tissue, this is referred to as heat and toxins.

Ingredients in the Formula:
Huang Lian (coptis rhizome) clears heat from the heart and from the digestive tract and is very effective in killing rod-shaped bacteria (bacilli) which are often

the cause of dysentery and diarrhea. It also calms irritability which is commonly found in many types of fever and illness and helps restore normal mental function.

Huang Qin (scutellaria root) clears extreme heat and toxins (bacterial infection) from the chest, stomach area and intestines. It reduces thick yellow phlegm and can be used to eliminate diarrhea and dysentery as well as reduce the symptoms of jaundice.

Huang Bai (phellodendron bark) clears heat from the lower part of the body and fights dysentery and diarrhea. It also helps fight urinary tract infections.

Zhi Zi (gardenia fruit) clears heat and toxins from liver and gallbladder, reduces irritability, restlessness and delirium. It also can be used to reduce swelling and heat from carbuncles, furuncles and boils.

Note: These pills can be ground into a powder and applied topically to any red, inflamed sore on the skin as long as it has not opened. It will reduce the swelling, heat and discomfort of most types of skin infections.

Modern laboratory research in China has shown that Huang Lian functions as a broad-spectrum antibiotic. It is effective in combating infections caused by various types of pathogenic bacteria including both gram-negative and gram-positive bacteria. It can reduce diplococci, streptococci, staphylococci, bacilli and spirilla including bacillus dysenteriae (dysentery), staphylococcus (skin infections, boils, carbuncles), streptococcus pneumoniae (bacterial pneumonia), Neisseria meningitidis (meningitis), corynebacterium diptheriae (diptheria), streptococcus (strep throat), mycobacterium tuberculosis (tuberculosis) and leptospira (hepatitis, jaundice).

Modern research has also demonstrated the antibiotic effects of the other herbs in this formula as well in treating fungal organisms, pathogenic tinea, trichomonas, and several other skin related conditions.

In addition, preparations of these herbs have proven to be effective in treating bacteria which have become resistant to pharmaceutical drugs such as streptomycin, chloramphenicol, and oxytetracycline hydrochloride.

Dosage: 3 pills three times per day.

HUANG LIAN SU WAN

Coptis Tea Pills
Modern Single-Herb Formula

Common Usage: Dysentery, diarrhea, traveler's diarrhea.

Description: Huang Lian Su is a concentrated form of the herb Huang Lian (coptis rhizome) which has been found to be a natural antibiotic. It kills the rod-shaped bacteria that are often found in contaminated food and water which cause traveler's diarrhea. It can also be used for acute watery stool or brief bloody diarrhea.

This medicine is popular in China and is often carried by travelers, along with Pill Curing or Po Chai Pills (see pages 223, 230), to treat minor cases of diarrhea which result from eating contaminated food.

Modern laboratory research in China has shown that Huang Lian functions as a broad-spectrum antibiotic. It is effective in combating infections caused by various types of pathogenic bacteria including both gram-negative and gram-positive bacteria. It can reduce diplococci, streptococci, staphylococci, bacilli and spirilla including bacillus dysenteriae (dysentery), staphylococcus (skin infections, boils, carbuncles), streptococcus pneumoniae (bacterial pneumonia), Neisseria meningitidis (meningitis), corynebacterium diptheriae (diptheria), streptococcus (strep throat), mycobacterium tuberculosis (tuberculosis) and leptospira (hepatitis, jaundice).

Dosage: 8 pills three times per day.

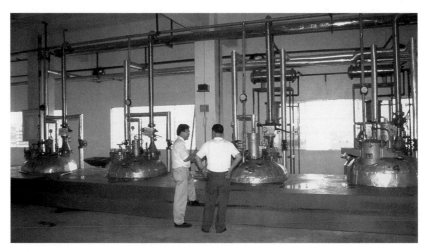

Cookers, Pangaoshou

JIA WEI XIAO YAO WAN

Extra Flavor Xiao Yao Wan
Dan Zhi Xiao Yao Wan
Free and Easy Wanderer Plus
Summary of Internal Medicine
(Nei Ke Zhai Yao)
Dr. Wen Sheng, Mid-19th Century

Common Usage: PMS, anger, irritability.

Description: Currently, one of the most popular Chinese herb formulas in the United States, Xiao Yao Wan (see page 116) is often taken by women in between the menses to eliminate the symptoms of PMS. These symptoms occur because of concurrent blood deficiency and emotional constriction of the liver which controls the free flow of blood. Xiao Yao Wan nourishes blood and helps to regulate the liver to promote the movement of Qi and blood in the body, reducing PMS symptoms.

The emotional symptoms of PMS—distress, upset and anxiety—are commonly looked upon by Western doctors as a psychosomatic condition. Symptoms of PMS include bloating, fatigue, headache, dizziness, blurry vision, dry mouth and throat. as well as reduced appetite and an irregular menstrual cycle that often includes cramps. All of these symptoms can be relieved by regular consumption of Xiao Yao Wan.

Jia Wei Xiao Yao Wan is an amended formulation of Xiao Yao Wan, with the addition of *Zhi Zi* (gardenia fruit) and *Mu Dan Pi* (moutan peony root bark) and is best suited for a woman with PMS, plus heat signs such as red face, night sweats, red eyes, or dry mouth. It is especially useful for those who experience anger, short temper or irritability because of PMS. The additional two herbs help the prescription by clearing the heat that causes irritability and anger, which in Chinese Medicine are always associated with some kind of internal heat.

Ingredients in the Formula:

Chai Hu (bupleurum root) relieves stagnation in the liver (constriction of emotions) and alleviates disharmony of the chest and stomach, controlling such symptoms as bloating, nausea and indigestion.

Bai Shao (white peony root) builds blood and relaxes the liver. This is extremely important for normal menstruation because the liver controls the flow of blood in the body. If there is constriction from stress or other reasons, the blood and Qi will not flow easily and menstruation will be difficult.

Dang Gui (angelica sinensis root) builds and regulates blood and, most importantly, controls contractions of the uterus, stopping cramps. Dang Gui is an important gynecological herb because it helps balance and harmonize the female organs.

Bai Zhu (atractylodes rhizome) improves digestion and assimilation of nutrients and thus helps to build healthier blood.

Bo He (mint herb) calms the emotions and addresses gynecological problems by soothing the liver and eliminating constraint brought about by stress.

Fu Ling (poria cocos fungus) improves digestion and drains excess fluids. It is very common for women to retain fluids just before their menses, and Fu Ling promotes urination to drain excess dampness. It also helps the other herbs to calm the emotions.

Gan Cao (licorice root) and *Sheng Jiang* (fresh ginger rhizome) harmonize the formula, improve digestion, and support lung function.

Zhi Zi (gardenia fruit) clears heat from the liver and gallbladder and is especially notable for removing irritability.

Mou Dan Pi (Moutan peony root bark) clears heat and cools the blood, calms the emotions and prevents stagnation. Whenever there is stagnation in the body, it leads to heat and pain. In Chinese Medicine, it is said that wherever there is pain, there is also stagnation. Remove the stagnation and the pain will go away. Mou Dan Pi also helps to prevent stagnation by moving the blood.

Dosage: 8 pills three times per day.

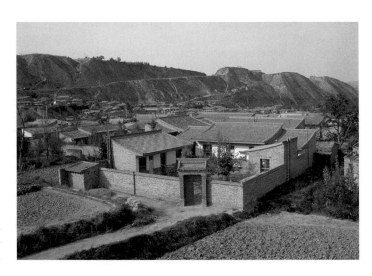

Village outside Lanzhou

167

JIN GU DIE SHENG WAN

Chin Koo Tieh Shang Wan
Muscle and Bone Trauma Pills
The Great Mender
[Based on: Die Da Wan]
Trauma Injury Pills
Collection of Chinese Herbal Prepared Medicines
(Quan Guo Zhong Cheng Yao Chu Fang Ji)
Author and Date Unknown

Common Usage: For minor sprains, strains, cuts, bruises and abrasions.

Description: This formula reduces pain, swelling and inflammation. It was designed primarily to help repair acute traumatic injury such as broken bones, muscle strains, knee and ankle strains. This prescription stops internal bleeding, reduces pain and helps to repair damage caused by many different types of injuries.

Chinese Diagnosis: Injury like this is called Die Da (punched by a blow). Many martial arts masters have concocted their own liniments and massage oils to treat bruises and injuries received during training. This formula comes from the martial arts tradition, but instead of being a topical treatment like a liniment, it is designed to be taken internally and is used to heal bruising, injury and wounds.

In Western Medicine, ice is almost always applied to injuries to reduce swelling and to reduce pain. In Chinese Medicine, this is not the case. Ice creates more stagnation and retards the healing process by reducing blood flow to the affected area. For thousands of years, Chinese doctors have advocated the use of herbs and warming treatments to invigorate blood in order to encourage the healing process. If ice is used at all, it would only be used for a few minutes following the injury to temporarily reduce inflammation. After that, treatment consists of warming the injured area to break up stagnation so that nutrients can freely flow to get to the injury to speed up the healing process.

My own experience with treating injuries has shown that ice impedes the healing process and prolongs the injured condition. Acupuncture is remarkably effective in treating many types of injuries such as sprained ankles, twisted knees and sore backs. I have treated individuals with a sprained ankle who have been on crutches for two weeks with no improvement. Most often only one acupuncture treatment is necessary to get them walking without crutches again.

Jin Gu Die Sheng Wan can also be used to promote healing by those who have broken bones in an accident. My experience has shown that people heal in half the expected time when treated with this formula combined with acupuncture.

Ingredients in the Formula:

Tian Qi (panax notoginseng root) is valuable for treating almost any type of injury (see Tian Qi Wan, page 183). It has a unique ability to stop bleeding and to remove stagnation of blood at the same time. It helps to reduce swelling and inflammation and can assist in stopping pain. It is effective following accidents involving broken bones, bruises, sprains and any type of traumatic injury.

Chi Shao (red peony root) and *Bai Shao* (white peony root) combine together to break up blood stagnation, reduce swelling and pain, and moderate the warmer herbs in this formula so that the blood does not move out of control. Bai Shao also produces more blood to replenish blood lost in bleeding injuries.

Tao Ren (peach kernel seeds) and *Hong Hua* (safflower) are commonly paired together to break up blood stagnation caused by injury and bruising and to encourage the healing process.

Ru Xiang (frankincense) and *Mo Yao* (myrrh) are paired substances that reduce swelling, break up stagnation and stop pain.

Jiang Huang (curcuma longa rhizome) stops pain and swelling in the shoulders and upper arms.

Mu Dan Pi (moutan peony root bark) reduces swelling and bruises, helps to move blood stagnation, and cools the warming properties of some hot herbs in this formula. It balances the temperature of the entire formula.

Su Mu (sappan wood), one of the main ingredients in all Die Da formulas, stops pain and swelling from falls, broken bones, bruises and sprains.

Gu Sui Bu (drynaria rhizome) promotes the healing of tendons and bones. The name Gu Sui Bu literally

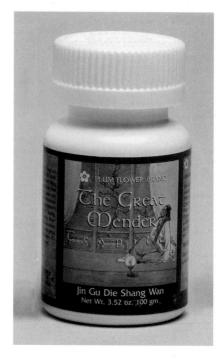

means "to mend broken bones." It is important for all simple fractures and injuries to tendons and ligaments.

San Leng (sparganium rhizome) breaks up blood stagnation, eliminates pain, and is often used in treating bruises, breaks, sprains, strains and other common injuries.

Xue Jie (daemonodrops resin), called Dragon's blood, breaks up blood stagnation and reduces pain, especially from injuries such as falls, fractures, contusions, sprains, strains and other trauma.

Liu Ji Nu (artemisia anomala herb) breaks up blood stagnation and reduces pain from trauma and injury, such as contusions, sprains, strains, falls and fractures.

Dang Gui (angelica sinensis root) invigorates blood and encourages the healing of wounds and injuries.

Xu Duan (dipsacus root) strengthens the lower back, knees and ankles by promoting the normal function of the liver and the kidneys.

Fang Feng (siler; ledebouriella root) reduces wind and dampness especially as they affect the skin surface of the body.

Tian Gua Zi (cucumis melon seed) reduces heat and inflammation.

Zhi Ke (aurantium fruit) breaks up Qi stagnation and reduces inflammation.

Gan Cao (licorice root) harmonizes the herbs in the formula.

Jie Geng (platycodon root) improves digestion and strengthens the lungs which carry healing energy to all areas of the body.

Mu Tong (akebia stem) drains dampness and therefore reduces inflammation and swelling.

Zi Ran Tong (pyrite) breaks up blood stagnation and heals broken bones, injured tendons, and reduces masses and inflammation.

Tu Bie Chong (eupolyphaga sinensis) breaks up blood stagnation, reduces masses and inflammation, strengthens tendons, heals contusions, lacerations and fractured bones.

Dosage: 8 pills three times per day.

NEI XIAO LUO LI WAN

Dissolve Internal Mass Pills
The Comprehensive Collection of Beneficial Treatments
(Yang Yi Da Quan)
Dr. Gu Shi-Cheng, Qing Dynasty 1644–1911 A.D.

Common Usage: Goiter, scrofula, neck tumors.

Description: This formula reduces swelling and clears abscesses where they most commonly form—on the neck and upper body. It can eliminate abscesses, sores that ulcerate, and inflamed infections, such as tubercular sores. It can also reduce the swelling of an enlarged thyroid gland (goiter).

In Chinese Medicine, when there is Qi stagnation, there will also be blood stagnation. Any time stagnation exists, the possibility of phlegm stagnation presents itself. Wherever there is stagnation, heat will manifest. Goiter is considered to be phlegm fire—phlegm stagnation which has grown hotter and hotter. Treatment of this condition is to increase blood circulation to the affected area. This will cool the heat, break up the stagnation and carry away the excess phlegm.

Ingredients in the Formula:

Xia Ku Cao (prunella vulgaris spike) clears heat and shrinks nodules, lumps and painful enlarged lymph glands, especially those that are red and inflamed.

Xuan Shen (scrophularia root) softens hard lumps, reduces nodules and clears heat from the throat.

Dang Gui (angelica sinensis root) increases blood flow to lumps and abscesses. Increased blood flow brings nutrients to assist the healing process and remove pus.

Mang Xiao (mirabilitum), *Da Huang* (rhubarb root) and *Gan Cao* (licorice root) are a three-herb formula called *Tiao Wei Cheng Qi Tang* (Regulate the Stomach and Order the Qi Formula). It clears heat in the bowels and purges constipation. This formula has been added to the larger formula to clear heat from the channels that traverse the neck and throat.

Zhi Ke (aurantium fruit) breaks up the stagnation of Qi. When Qi is congested, it blocks the flow of blood and phlegm which make up the substance of a mass or goiter. It also breaks up phlegm stagnation which blocks the free flow of Qi.

Zhe Bei Mu (fritillaria thunbergii bulb) and *Tian Hua Fen* (trichosanthes root) break up phlegm nodules on the upper part of the body.

Jie Geng (platycodon root) directs the energy of the prescription to the upper body, neck and throat, dissolves phlegm and heat, and expels pus.

171

Lian Qiao (forsythia fruit) expels heat and pus from accumulation under the skin. It heals sores and removes lumps.

Sheng Di Huang (raw rehmannia root) clears heat and cools blood, and it produces fluids to promote the healing of the body.

Bo He (mint herb) cools the throat and assists the liver to promote the free flow of blood which will in turn assist the healing of a mass.

Hai Zao (sargasso pallidum seaweed) helps to normalize the function of the thyroid. It promotes the healing of goiter and scrofula, breaking up the stagnation of phlegm and blood which enlarge the thyroid gland.

Qing Yan (halitium salt) cools blood and increases vasodilation to heal abscesses.

Bai Lian (ampelopsis japonica herb) is anti-inflammatory, anodyne, and cooling.

Hai Fen (notarchus leachii egg)

Gan Cao (licorice root) harmonizes the herbs in the formula.

Dosage: 8 pills three times per day.

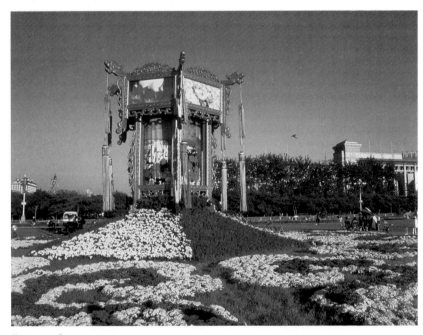

Tiananmen Square

NING SOU WAN

Stop Cough Pills
Quiet Cough
[Based on: Er Chen Wan]
[Two Good Old Herb Decoction]
Imperial Grace Formulary of the Tai Ping Era
(Tai Ping Hui Min He Ji Ju Fang)
Imperial Medicine Department, 1078–1085 A.D.

Common Usage: Stops cough, clears phlegm, stops wheezing.

Description: Ning Sou Wan stops cough by regulating and nourishing the lungs. It clears accumulated phlegm and directs the energy of the lungs downward so that the body can effectively utilize oxygen. It is a broad-spectrum formula which clears lung heat, stops wheezing (asthma), drains dampness which could be aggravating the cough, regulates the normal functions of the lungs and strengthens the function of the lungs.

In Chinese Medicine, the throat and bronchials are considered to be part of the lung system. When addressing a problem such as a cough, the lungs are likely to be affected as well as the throat.

Ingredients in the Formula:

Jie Geng (platycodon root) soothes the throat, expels phlegm and normalizes lung function. It helps to clear heat which can dry the lungs and cause cough.

Shi Hu (dendrobium herb) produces fluids to nourish dry lungs, helps dry mouth and throat, and eliminates thirst.

Er Chen Wan (see page 71)—*Ban Xia* (pinellia rhizome), *Ju Hong* (citrus orange peel), *Fu Ling* (poria cocos fungus) and *Gan Cao* (licorice root)—is a basic variation of the four-herb formula which clears phlegm and dampness from the lungs and helps to normalize lung function.

Chuan Bei Mu (fritillaria cirrhosa bulb) clears heat which can cause a dry cough and can be used when the lungs are weak and need to be tonified.

Bo He (mint herb) clears lung heat, cools the throat and stops cough. It also calms the liver which can disrupt the normal function of the lungs.

Zi Su Zi (perilla seed) and *Xing Ren* (apricot kernel) stop wheezing (asthma) and direct lung Qi downwards so that it will not disrupt normal breathing and cause a cough. They also lubricate the intestines, making it ideal for those with a cough plus constipation. In Chinese Medicine, there is an internal connection between the lungs and the large intestine. If the large intestine is constipated, the lung can be adversely affected.

Sang Bai Pi (mulberry root bark) stops coughing and wheezing.

Gu Ya (rice sprout) breaks up food stagnation in the digestive tract and helps to eliminate phlegm stagnation before it accumulates in the lungs or nasal passages.

Dosage: 8 pills three times per day.

PING WEI WAN

Calm Stomach Powder Pills
Move and Dry the Earth
Imperial Grace Formulary of the Tai Ping Era
(Tai Ping Hui Min He Ji Ju Fang)
Imperial Medical Department, 1078–1085 A.D.

Common Usage: Improves digestion.

Description: Often in summer, people consume many cold drinks and other cold foods, such as ice cream and sodas, which interfere with normal digestion. Cold and dampness often work together to create sluggishness in the bowels, harming the ability of the body to function properly. Symptoms of this condition can include nausea, vomiting, loss of appetite, bloating, loose stool and fatigue. It can also create a loss of taste in the mouth.

This is a more common problem in Southern China where there is a great deal of humidity which contributes to internal dampness in the body.

Ingredients in the Formula:
Cang Zhu (atractylodes lancea rhizome) dries dampness in the digestive system, strengthens the functions of the stomach and spleen, stops bloating, nausea, vomiting and improves appetite.

Hou Po (magnolia bark) regulates and helps to remove cold and dampness that clog digestion. The accumulation of cold and dampness causes stagnation of Qi in the digestive tract, blocking the normal downward movement of food in the intestines. This can cause bloating and fullness, the painful, unpleasant feeling of being "stuffed" after a meal. The combination of Cang Zhu and Hou Po clear the dampness and cold, harmonizing digestion.

Chen Pi (aged citrus peel) regulates the digestive system which includes functions of the liver, gallbladder, pancreas, duodenum, stomach and spleen. Chen Pi directs the digestive energy downward, stops bloating, belching and the uncomfortable feeling of fullness after a meal. It also dries dampness and helps to clear phlegm from the lungs. This is an important function because too much dampness clogging the digestion can lead to phlegm accumulation in the lungs. In Chinese Medicine, it is said that the spleen creates dampness and the lungs store it.

Sheng Jiang (fresh ginger rhizome) warms the digestive fire, improves breathing which may be affected by the accumulation of cold and dampness in the lungs, and harmonizes the digestive system.

Gan Cao (licorice root) and *Da Zao* (black jujube dates) harmonize and improve digestion.

Dosage: 8 pills three times per day.

SANG JU YIN WAN
Mulberry Leaf and Chrysanthemum Drink Pills
Clear Wind-Heat Pills
Systematic Differentiation of Warm Diseases
(Wen Bing Tiao Bian)
Dr. Wu Ju-Tong, 1798 A.D.

Common Usage: Common cold, especially in children.

Description: Sang Ju Yin Wan is intended to treat common colds. It is especially good for children because it is mild and because children are more likely to have complications along with a cold. In this case, Sang Ju Yin Wan can be taken in situations where a common cold in very early stages is accompanied by red eyes or a headache with sore throat and fever.

This formula is only effective in the early stages of cold or flu. It is most effective when taken within two or three days of the onset of the cold. If a cold persists beyond two or three days or seems to be going into the lungs, you should choose a different formula or see a licensed acupuncturist.

Sang Ju Yin is a variation of Yin Qiao San (see pages 121, 214), containing many of the same herbs. The difference between Sang Ju Yin and Yin Qiao San is that Sang Ju Yin is more gentle and can be taken by children. Also, Sang Ju Yin treats a common cold accompanied by cough, headache or red eyes.

Ingredients in the Formula:

Sang Ye (mulberry leaf) cools heat in the lungs and reduces fever, red eyes and sore throat.

Ju Hua (chrysanthemum flower) treats heat conditions which affect the head, such as headache and red, irritated eyes.

Lian Qiao (forsythia fruit) clears heat and fights infections in the fashion of an antibiotic, reducing fever, clearing sore throat and relieving headache.

Xing Ren (apricot seed) stops coughing and wheezing, directs the oxygen down into the lungs and relieves constipation which often accompanies fever conditions.

Jie Geng (platycodon root) helps nourish the lungs, stops cough and sore throat. It also aids digestion which generally improves the body's immune system.

Bo He (mint herb) clears heat from the head, relieving headache, sore throat and cough.

Lu Gen (phragmites communis rhizome) clears heat in the stomach and lungs. When there is heat in the lungs, it is difficult to breathe and rising heat can create a cough. Lu Gen not only clears heat from the lungs, but it also promotes fluids to moisten the lungs and the throat. Fluids are often burned up by a fever, and Lu Gen replenishes those lost fluids.

Gan Cao (licorice root) harmonizes the herbs in the formula.

Dosage: 8 pills three times per day.

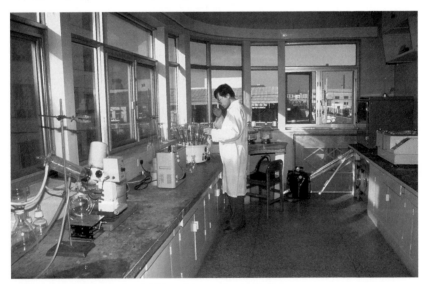

Quality control lab, Tianjin Great Wall Brand Factory, Free Trade Zone

SHENG MAI SAN

Generate the Pulse Powder Pills
The Great Pulse
Clarifying Doubts about Injury from Internal and External Causes
(Nei Wai Shang Bian Huo Lun)
Dr. Li Ao, 1247 A.D.

Common Usage: Chronic cough, fatigue, debility.

Description: This prescription restores the energy which drives the pulse. It is meant to restore and strengthen a weak constitution which generates a weak pulse. It also helps to replenish fluids which have been lost from excessive sweating. It promotes both Qi and Yin (body fluids). Often taken when sweating excessively in summer, this formula is used to treat those who are tired, thirsty and dizzy.

Ingredients in the Formula:

Ren Shen (panax ginseng root) is the strongest herb to restore strength and power to an exhausted individual. It rebuilds basic, fundamental energy which can show up as shortness of breath, difficulty breathing, a lack of appetite and severe fatigue.

Mai Men Dong (ophiopogonis tuber) cools internal body heat and restores fluids. It also assists the lungs, stops dry cough, dry mouth and dry tongue. It calms irritability and restores emotional harmony.

Wu Wei Zi (schisandra fruit) strengthens the lungs to improve breathing and stops sweating. It also calms the restless heart and the mind.

Dosage: 8 pills three times per day.

SI JUN ZI TANG WAN

Four Gentlemen
Imperial Grace Formulary of the Tai Ping Era
(Tai Ping Hui Min He Ji Ju Fang)
Imperial Medical Department, 1078–1085 A.D.

Common Usage: Improves digestion, strengthens the immune system.

Description: Four Gentlemen formula is the single most important herb formula in all of Chinese Medicine for improving digestion. It is the foundation for almost all prescriptions directed toward nourishing the spleen. Without healthy digestion, individuals do not sustain good health or recover well from illness.

Chinese Diagnosis: According to tradition, many diseases are the direct result of digestive weakness. The Chinese call digestive weakness spleen deficiency. The spleen includes the digestive functions of the liver, gallbladder, pancreas, duodenum, stomach and spleen. Spleen deficiency indicates that the patient is not getting appropriate nutrients from the food he or she eats. Without the good Qi from food, the body cannot build good blood and the cells do not receive the nourishment they need to replicate and prosper.

The main symptoms of spleen deficiency are bloating, loose stool, fatigue and low appetite. Other symptoms include weak arms and legs, pale complexion, skinny, and undeveloped muscles. These symptoms can be seen in those who don't get enough to eat or in those who don't assimilate the food that they do eat.

Generally, a doctor of Chinese Medicine would include this formula or a variation of it in a larger prescription for any patient who is spleen deficient, but it can be taken alone and long term because it is a relatively gentle treatment. It can be used by almost anyone who experiences digestive problems.

Digestive problems, including gastrointestinal disease, are the number one complaint of patients in the United States. Western Medicine offers no treatment for digestive complaints other than antacids, ulcer medications, drugs to kill parasites and laxatives. Chinese Medicine, on the other hand, provides literally hundreds of treatments for various types of digestive difficulties, many of which help to promote normal function. This is just one of them.

Ingredients in the Formula:

Ren Shen (panax ginseng root) strengthens the spleen Qi and increases the body's overall energy. If digestion can be improved, more nutrients can be extracted from food and can be utilized by the body. When digestion is healthy, other bodily functions will also remain healthy or improve. Ren Shen also fortifies the lungs and improves breathing which allows for improved consumption of oxygen and therefore better energy.

Bai Zhu (atractylodes rhizome) warms the digestive fire which cooks food and dries dampness that accumulates when digestion isn't working well. Accumulation of dampness causes stagnation in the bowels, clogs up the lungs, bronchials and mucus membranes and interferes with normal breathing and digestion.

Fu Ling (poria cocos fungus) drains dampness from the digestive system and strengthens spleen Qi. It directs fluids to the right places in the body and clears fluid from areas where it shouldn't accumulate.

Gan Cao (licorice root) harmonizes the herbs in this prescription, directs the Qi into all parts of the body and improves the function of the lungs.

Dosage: 8 pills three times per day.

SI WU TANG WAN

Four Substances
Imperial Grace Formulary of the Tai Ping Era
(Tai Ping Hui Min He Ji Ju Fang)
Imperial Medical Department, 1078–1085 A.D.

Common Usage: Anemia, normalize menses.

Description: One of the most fundamental formulas in all of Chinese Medicine, Si Wu Tang is the foundation for many women's formulas because it nourishes and regulates blood, treating anemia and normalizing the menstrual cycle.

The symptoms of blood deficiency include blurry vision, dizziness, pale face and an irregular menstrual cycle. The irregular menstrual cycle can include little or no blood flow during menses, painful and difficult menstrual cycle, and other menstrual difficulties.

Ingredients in the Formula:
Dang Gui (angelica sinensis root) nourishes and regulates blood. It is the main herb in Chinese Medicine to assist women both with hormones and with blood. It helps to stop cramps before, during and after menses. In this century there have been a large number of studies regarding Dang Gui, documenting its positive effects on the function of the uterus.

Shu Di Huang (prepared rehmannia root) nourishes blood to eliminate anemia. It also helps replenish yin body fluids which include hormones which are carried by the blood. Shu Di Huang strengthens the kidneys and helps prevent lower back pain and gray hair.

Bai Shao (white peony root) nourishes blood, stops pain, cramps and spasms. It helps to eliminate cramps by promoting the production of more blood and by helping the body to retain vital fluids which lubricate muscles, tendons and bones. Bai Shao is also an important herb to help normalize the liver function which controls blood flow during the menstrual cycle.

Chuan Xiong (ligusticum root) regulates blood, moves stagnant blood, and stops pain, cramps and headache. It is a very important herb in gynecological conditions.

Dosage: 8 pills three times a day.

TAO HONG SI WU TANG WAN

Peach Kernel and Safflower Plus Four Substance Formula Pills
Golden Mirror of the Medical Tradition
(Yi Zong Jin Jian)
Dr. Wu Qian, 1742 A.D.

Special Warning: This product should not be taken by women with normal or heavy blood flow because it could cause excessive bleeding. It should be discontinued once menses starts because it could cause excessive loss of blood, unless clots are very large or the menses stops mid cycle.

Common Usage: Regulates menses, eliminates clotting.

Description: Tao Hong Si Wu Tang Wan would be used for blood stagnation and blood deficiency. This formula is designed for a woman who is having very painful cramps just before menses or during the first day or two of the cycle, possibly including purple dark clots. It could be for a woman whose period starts then stops and starts again due to stagnant blood.

Ingredients in the Formula:

Dang Gui (angelica sinensis root) nourishes and regulates blood. It is important in assisting women both with hormones and with blood.

Shu Di Huang (prepared rehmannia root) nourishes blood to eliminate anemia. It also helps replenish yin body fluids which include hormones.

Bai Shao (white peony root) nourishes blood, stops pain, cramps and spasms. It helps to eliminate cramps by promoting the production of more blood and by helping the body to retain vital fluids which lubricate muscles, tendons and bones. Bai Shao is also an important herb to help normalize the liver function which controls blood flow during the menstrual cycle.

Chuan Xiong (ligusticum root) regulates blood, and helps stop pain, cramps and headache. It is a very important gynecological herb.

Hong Hua (safflower) and Tao Ren (peach kernel) break up blood stagnation and stops clotting.

Dosage: 8 pills three times per day.

TIAN MA GOU TENG WAN
Gastrodia and Uncaria Pills
New Significance of Patterns and Treatment in Miscellaneous Diseases
(Za Bing Zheng Zhi Xin Yi)
Author and Date Unknown

Common Usage: High blood pressure, headache, muscle spasms.

Description: This formula treats hypertension (high blood pressure) and other associated symptoms, such as migraine headache, muscle spasms, shaking and/or red eyes, blurry vision, dizziness, deafness, ear ringing, anger, irritability and stiff tongue.

Chinese Diagnosis: All of these symptoms are possible manifestations of a condition of underlying liver and kidney Yin deficiency with liver Yang rising and internal movement of liver wind. When the liver blood is insufficient, it cannot properly lubricate the muscles and tendons. When muscles and tendons are dry, they will spasm and twitch. Any unnatural movement of the body or of body parts, such as twitching, deviation of the tongue or eyes, is called liver wind.

In each individual, there is always a balance between yin fluids and yang energy. When the yin fluids are too low, the body becomes imbalanced. As in nature, when there is not enough water to control a fire, the fire will flare upward and grow out of control. In this case, the yin water cannot control the yang fire which rises upward to affect the head, causing ear ringing, shaking eyes, deafness and headache.

A number of the herbs in this formula have been shown by modern research to lower blood pressure.

When there is an excess of cholesterol, fat deposits build up in the blood and coat the vessels walls, shrinking the lumen through which the blood flows. When there is less space for the blood, the pressure inside the vessels increases.

People who are overweight often have high blood pressure. This herb formula is beneficial for them because it reduces edema (excess water), thereby lowering blood pressure.

This formula clears heat from the liver, calms the mind, eliminates wind and nourishes the liver and kidneys.

Ingredients in the Formula:
Tian Ma (gastrodia rhizome) and *Gou Teng* (uncaria stem) extinguish internal wind, stop spasms and reduce irritability. Tian Ma is especially helpful in eliminating dizziness, headaches and pain. Gou Teng has been proven in clinical tests to lower blood pressure.

Niu Xi (achyranthes root) pulls energy downward from the head, nourishes tendons and bones. Nu Xi has proven in clinical exams to lower blood pressure.

Du Zhong (eucommia bark) strengthens the liver and the kidneys and promotes proper circulation of blood. It can also be taken for lower back pain, sore, weak knees and frequent urination. It also lowers blood pressure.

Fu Ling (poria cocos fungus) calms the spirit, aids digestion and helps to nourish internal organs by improving digestion and expediting the proper movement of fluids in the body.

Ye Jiao Teng (polygonum multiflorium vine) helps to soften tendons by nourishing blood. It also calms the spirit.

Sang Ji Sheng (mulberry parasite) reduces the symptoms of arthritis and has been proven in clinical tests to lower blood pressure.

Yi Mu Cao (leonurus; Chinese motherwort leaf) reduces swelling and masses, breaking up stagnation in the blood.

Huang Qin (scutellaria root) clears heat from the upper part of the body, calming excess liver yang which can create headaches, red eyes and a feeling of heat in the face. Huang Qin also lowers blood pressure.

Zhi Zi (gardenia fruit) controls heat in the liver and gallbladder. Liver heat is a common condition created by stress and congested emotions. When emotions constrict the liver, the blood and Qi do not flow freely. As with a radiator, if there is restricted movement, heat increases. Physics teaches that heat always rises. In the case of the human body, heat rises to the head and causes the previously discussed problems. Zhi Zi lowers blood pressure.

Dosage: 8 pills three times per day.

TIAN QI WAN

Notoginseng Pills
Modern Single-Herb Formula

Special Warning: For serious, life-threatening traumatic injuries, please go to the nearest hospital.

Common Usage: Stops bleeding, eases pain from trauma and injury.

Description: This product can be taken any time after minor injuries, including bruising, abrasions, minor accidents and other trauma. It helps to stop internal bleeding and to ease pain.

Tian Qi powder is found in many topical oils, creams and liniments. These products are often used by martial arts masters to treat injuries like sprains, strains and bruises sustained during practice.

It has been reported that Viet Cong and North Vietnamese soldiers during the Viet Nam war carried Tian Qi powder with them at all times to apply to wounds and to stop bleeding from gun shots. In Asia, this herb is widely used for all types of injuries, cuts, contusions, broken bones and other trauma.

Note: The pills can be ground into powder and sprinkled on the affected area in order to help heal wounds, small cuts, and abrasions. It can also be applied topically to stop bleeding on any open wound.

Dosage: 8 pills three times per day.

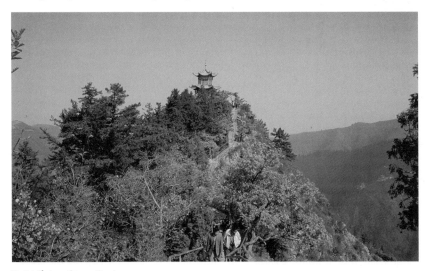

Taoist Shrine, Giansu Province

TONG JING WAN

Regulate the Menses Pills
Calm in the Sea of Life
The English-Chinese Encyclopedia of
Practical Traditional Chinese Medicine, Vol. #5
Chief Editor Xu Xiang-Cai, 1989 A.D.

Special Warning: This prescription should not be used by women who are pregnant (it could induce an abortion or miscarriage) or by women who are extremely anemic or blood deficient. Any woman with a pale face with a pale tongue who is often late starting her period or has short, scanty periods with pale blood should not use this product.

Common Usage: Regulates difficult menstruation.

Description: At times, many women experience difficult menstruation. It is not uncommon for a woman to find that her menstrual period is late. This can be caused by blood stagnation that keeps the blood from flowing normally. Tong Jing Wan breaks up blood stagnation and induces menstruation.

Chinese Diagnosis: A late period can be caused by many different factors, one of the most common of which is constrained emotions. Constrained emotions affect the free flow of liver Qi, causing the blood to stagnate. Blood clots are evidence of congealed stagnant blood. This prescription breaks up clots and encourages the free flow of blood.

It can be used by any woman who is late or who experiences cramps, purple or dark clots, and an irregular period with dark blood.

Ingredients in the Formula:

Tao Ren (peach kernel) and *Hong Hua* (safflower) are paired herbs that break up blood stagnation. They have very strong actions to induce blood flow. Research in China indicates that Hong Hua stimulates contractions of the uterus.

Bai Shao (white peony root) cools heat in the liver that may be causing stagnation. Modern research has shown that Bai Shao is anti-inflammatory and stops muscle spasms.

Dan Shen (salvia root) cools the blood, eases irritability and soothes the liver which often affects emotions and the menstrual cycle.

Pu Huang (typhae pollen) stops pain and ensures that there will not be excessive bleeding. It boasts the unique characteristics of moving blood, breaking up stagnation and stopping bleeding. Modern research has shown that Pu Huang has a strong stimulating effect on the uterus.

Wu Yao (lindera root) stops menstrual pain, warms the womb and supports the kidneys. This is especially effective when internal cold blocks the menstrual function.

Yan Hu Suo (corydalis rhizome) stops pain, especially in the lower abdomen, and is very effective with symptoms of dysmennorhea or difficult menses and cramps. Modern research from China proves that Yan Hu Suo has analgesic properties and stops pain due to difficult menstruation.

Dang Gui (angelica sinensis root) is the single most important herb in gynecology. It nourishes blood, moves blood and helps reduce pain. Modern research indicates that Dang Gui has a strong effect on the normal functioning of the uterus.

Chuan Xiong (ligusticum root) regulates the menstrual cycle, moving both blood and Qi, and otherwise normalizing menstrual function. Research in China indicates that Chuan Xiong has a stimulating effect on the uterus.

Xiang Fu (cyperus rhizome) regulates the free flow of liver Qi which has a powerful influence on the normal function of the menstrual cycle.

Tian Qi (panax notoginseng root) moves blood and stops abnormal bleeding, again ensuring that bleeding will not be excessive. It has anti-inflammatory properties and stops abdominal pain.

Dosage: 8 pills three times per day.

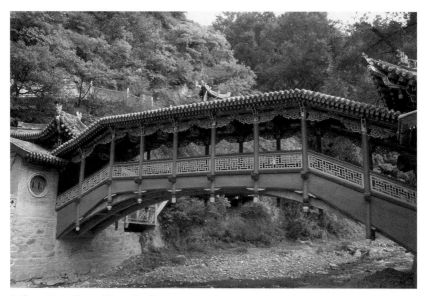

Bridge to Taoist Shrine, Giansu Province

TONG SHUN WAN

Flow Through Smoothly Pills
Discussion of Spleen and Stomach
(Pi Wei Lun)
Dr. Li Dong-Yuan, 1249 A.D.

Common Usage: Laxative.

Description: This formula is a very strong laxative, containing not only seeds which lubricate the intestines, but also two strong purgative herbs—Da Huang and Fan Xie Ye. This formula should only be taken by individuals for whom other laxatives are ineffective.

Ingredients in the Formula:
Tao Ren (peach seed) and *Huo Ma Ren* (marijuana seed) contain oil that lubricates the intestines. Tao Ren also breaks up stagnation in the intestines, and Huo Ma Ren produces more yin fluids which soften the stool.

Qian Hu (peucedanum root) directs lung energy down and resolves sticky phlegm. In Chinese Medicine, there is a close association between the lungs and the large intestine. When the lung Qi is stuck, it often affects the normal downward direction of the intestines. If energy is stuck above, it may also be stuck below. This herb normalizes lung energy and encourages downward flow.

Dang Gui (angelica sinensis root) nourishes blood and also helps the movement of blood. This combination produces fluids to soften the stool and helps to break up stagnation that may impact feces in the intestines.

Da Huang (rhubarb root) is a strong purgative.

Fan Xie Ye (senna leaf), another purgative, is often used by older people whose intestines have weakened and do not have strong peristaltic action to move the stool..

Dosage: 6 pills once per day.

WEN JING TANG WAN

Warm the Menses Pills
Warm Cycle
Essentials of the Golden Cabinet
(Jin Gui Yao Lue)
Dr. Chang Chung-Ching, 142–220 A.D.

Special Warning: Do not use during pregnancy.

Common Usage: Infertility, irregular menstruation.

Description: This formula treats menstrual irregularity. This is a case of cold obstructing the lower abdomen which may cause a woman to feel that her lower abdomen is cold. There may be irregular menses, either early or late, excessive or scant blood flow, blood clots which would be purple in color, bleeding between periods, infertility, dry lips and mouth, and cold hands and feet.

It is also possible that a woman could have both hot and cold symptoms, indicating that her body is not properly balanced. It can be caused by a hormone imbalance or menopausal symptoms. It can also be caused by yin fluids and yang fire both being deficient at the same time--heat above and cold below.

Ingredients in the Formula:

This formula contains *Si Wu Tang Wan* (Four Substances Formula; see page 179) as its foundation: *Dang Gui* (angelica sinensis root), *Chuan Xiong* (ligusticum root), *Bai Shao* (white peony root) and *Shu Di Huang* (prepared rehmannia root). One of the most fundamental formulas in all of Chinese Medicine, Si Wu Tang is the basis for many women's prescriptions because it nourishes and regulates blood, treating anemia and normalizing the menstrual cycle.

Ren Shen (panax ginseng root), *Sheng Jiang* (fresh ginger root) and *Gan Cao* (licorice root) all help to improve digestion and energy.

Wu Zhu Yu (evodia fruit) warms the lower abdomen, stops pain and unblocks cold stagnation in the liver channel which wraps around the genitals.

Gui Zhi (cinnamon twig) opens the channels and unblocks cold, stagnant blood that affects the menses. It also sends warming energy to the hands and feet.

Mu Dan Pi (moutan peony root bark) clears heat from the blood and moves blood stagnation from excess heat. It is commonly used in gynecological prescriptions to eliminate liver blood stagnation that may be affecting the normal period.

Mai Men Dong (ophiopogonis tuber) cools heat and nourishes yin body fluids that include hormones.

Ban Xia (pinellia rhizome) regulates digestion, dries dampness and breaks up phlegm stagnation.

Dosage: 8 pills three times per day.

WU PI YIN WAN

Five Peel Powder Pills
Treasury Classic
(Zhong Zang Jing)
Dr. Hua Tuo, Six Dynasties Period

Caution: No diuretic should be taken long term.

Common Usage: Diuretic.

Description: Five Skin Pills are a combination of herbs designed to treat edema and to eliminate water retention. It is especially useful in treating edema that collects on the surface of the body, such as superficial facial edema. This is a gentle herb formula and can be taken for any type of edema or water retention.

The symptoms of edema are water retention, swelling, a feeling of overall heaviness, a sense of distention, fullness in the chest or abdomen, difficult breathing, and perhaps urinary difficulty.

Ingredients in the Formula:

Fu Ling Pi (poria cocos fungus skin) drains dampness more strongly than the herb, Fu Ling, from which the skin, Fu Ling Pi, is derived.

Sang Bai Pi (mulberry root bark) encourages urination by promoting the downward flow of Qi in the body. It clears edema, especially on the face, hands and feet.

Chen Pi (aged citrus peel) regulates Qi, breaks up phlegm stagnation and normalizes the functions of the stomach and digestive system which control the processing of water in the body.

Sheng Jiang Pi (fresh ginger root skin) drains dampness and reduces edema.

Ze Xie Pi (alisma rhizome peel) clears heat and promotes urination which drains dampness from the body, eliminating edema.

Bai Bian Dou (dolichos seed) improves digestion which is often responsible for retention of fluids.

Dosage: 8 pills three times per day.

WU REN WAN

Five Seed Pills
Effective Formulas from Generations of Physicians
(Shi Yi De Xiao Fang)
Dr. Wei Yi-Lin, 1345 A.D.

Common Usage: Laxative.

Description: Five Seed Pills contain five different seeds which lubricate the intestines and encourage bowel movement. This formula is especially beneficial to the elderly whose body fluids have dried up. Unlike Ma Zi Ren Wan, which clears heat and lubricates, this formula simply moistens the intestines and helps to normalize the downward function of digestion.

Ingredients in the Formula:

Xing Ren (apricot kernel) lubricates the intestines and promotes the downward movement of Qi.

Tao Ren (peach kernel) lubricates intestines and breaks up stagnation.

Bai Zi Ren (biota seed) calms the mind, promotes liver blood, and lubricates the intestines.

Yu Li Ren (prunus japonica seed) lubricates intestines and works as a mild purgative to encourage peristaltic action and bowel movement.

Song Zi Ren (pine nut) lubricates the intestines.

Chen Pi (aged citrus peel) regulates digestion and normalizes the downward flow of Qi in the intestines. It helps to prevent the possible stagnation of the oily substances in the intestines.

Dosage: 6 pills three times per day.

WU WEI XIAO DU YIN WAN

Five Flavors to Clear Toxins Drink Pills
Golden Mirror of the Medical Tradition
(Yi Zong Jin Jian)
Dr. Wu Qian, 1742 A.D.

Special Warning: See a licensed practitioner when treating any lesion on the skin or any lump under the skin. It is important to have a correct diagnosis and to be certain that it isn't potentially serious.

Common Usage: Boils, carbuncles, skin swelling, infected acne.

Description: This formula treats boils, carbuncles, or any skin swelling that is hard, red and painful. It must be used before the swelling has erupted and before it has started to weep. These herbs are combined together in order to clear the heat and toxins that have accumulated beneath the skin. It can be taken orally in pill form, or the pills can be crushed, made into a paste, and applied directly on the swelling.

Chinese Diagnosis: Boils or carbuncles often occur after a sickness with fever or from very hot summer conditions. A diet of rich, greasy, spicy foods makes an individual especially susceptible. The heat generated internally from spicy foods creates stagnation which is affected by external heat and dampness, aggravating the underlying condition. Boils or lesions move to the surface to expel the accumulation of heat, dampness and toxins.

Ingredients in the Formula:

Jin Yin Hua (honeysuckle flower; lonicera japonicas) is important in clearing heat and fighting infections that accumulate under the skin.

Pu Gong Ying (dandelion herb) is very important for its natural antibiotic effects. It eliminates abscesses and firm, hard lumps under the skin.

Zi Hua Di Ding (viola yeodensis flower) heals sores and abscesses, especially on the head and back.

Ye Ju Hua (wild chrysanthemum flower) directs the healing energy to the surface of the skin and upward to the face and neck. It provides direction, heat reduction and removal of toxins.

Lian Qiao (forsythia fruit) reduces swelling, clears heat and toxins. It can be used for any skin condition with swelling, heat and pain such as poison oak, boils or any red, inflamed lump under the skin.

Note: If the skin has erupted and there is an open sore or pus is oozing out, this formula is no longer appropriate.

It is possible to make a poultice or paste of the herbs in this formula and apply to the skin. The herbs can be purchased in any Chinese herb shop, or they can be ordered from any of a number of companies that provide mail order service. See resource list at the back of this book.

Dosage: 8 pills three times per day.

XIANG LIAN WAN

Aucklandia and Coptis Pills
Imperial Grace Formulary of the Tai Ping Era
(Tai Ping Hui Min He Ji Ju Fang)
Imperial Medical Department, 1078–1085 A.D.

Common Usage: Stops diarrhea, regulates digestion.

Description: For treatment of diarrhea, red (blood) and white (mucus) diarrhea, abdominal pain, burning anus.

Ingredients in the Formula:
Huang Lian (coptis rhizome) kills almost all rod-shaped bacteria that cause diarrhea (see Huang Lian Su Wan, pages 165, 235).

Mu Xiang (saussurea root) regulates the intestines and helps to normalize the function of the bowels and digestion.

Dosage: 8 pills three times per day.

XIAO HUO LUO DAN

Small Opening the Channels Pills
Imperial Grace Formulary of the Tai Ping Era
(Tai Ping Hui Min He Ji Ju Fang)
Imperial Medical Department, 1078–1085 A.D.

Special Warning: This formula should never be taken by anyone with heat signs, such as a rapid pulse, red face, inflamed joints or a red tongue. The herbs in this formula are very warming and will aggravate heat conditions. It should not be taken during pregnancy.

Common Usage: Paralysis, arthritis, post-stroke.

Description: All three of the above conditions occur as the result of channel blockage. These channels, also called meridians and collaterals, can become blocked for a number of reasons.

Arthritis, usually damp and cold stagnation, impedes the normal flow of energy through the meridians, restricting movement and causing pain in the joints. Arthritis is often associated with numbness, pain, stiff joints and difficulty of movement.

A stroke blocks the free flow of Qi in the meridians and most often restricts the flow of blood in the vessels. When blood and Qi are blocked from moving freely, pain usually results. Tissues are not nourished properly, atrophy, and become numb to sensation.

Chinese Diagnosis: This formula opens up the meridians and blood vessels to promote the free flow of Qi and blood in the body, especially in the legs and lower back, thus contributing to enhanced mobility and increased sensation.

Ingredients in the Formula:

Chuan Wu (aconite carmichaeli) and *Fu Zi* (prepared aconite) are very hot herbs that warm the channels and open the vessels. They warm yang Qi, the vital life force energy that propels the body, and drive out cold and dampness.

Di Long (lumbricus; dried earthworm) opens the channels and meridians, improves the flexibility and range of motion in stiff joints, and eliminates paralysis. It is especially useful after a stroke because it has the ability to stop muscle spasms.

Dan Nan Xing (prepared arisaema) dissolves phlegm and removes blockage in the channels. It is common in strokes for plaque and cholesterol to break off in a blood vessel and flow into the brain where it clogs arteries and cuts off blood circulation. Dan Nan Xing dissolves the phlegm stagnation that is clogging the vessel.

Ru Xiang (frankincense) and *Mo Yao* (myrrh) are paired herbs that invigorate blood and stop pain. Together they encourage the free flow of yang Qi and reduce rigidity and stiffness.

Note: In the original loose herb formula, this prescription was taken with warm rice wine to increase the formula's ability to invigorate Qi and blood.

Dosage: 6 pills three times per day.

XIAO JIAN ZHONG WAN
Minor Restore the Middle Pills
Discussion of Cold-induced Disorders
(Shang Han Lun)
Dr. Chang Chung-Ching, 142–220 A.D.

Common Usage: Ulcers, stomach pain.

Description: Xiao Jian Zhong Wan warms and nourishes the digestive system. It also harmonizes the internal organs to reduce discomfort and pain as well as to balance the protective mechanism of the body to prevent colds and sickness. It protects by improving digestion which then makes nutrients more readily available to strengthen the protective Qi of the body.

Chinese Diagnosis: It can be taken when an individual has abdominal pain that is relieved by warmth. It is ideal for someone whose discomfort is relieved by pressing something hot or warm against the stomach. A stomach ulcer is often caused by overwork, improper eating habits, or poor diet and leads to a deficiency of middle (spleen and stomach) Qi, creating a hospitable environment for the lesion.

Ingredients in the Formula:
Bai Shao (white peony root) nourishes blood, elevating the white blood cell count to fight infections. It also helps stop pain in the stomach and intestines.

Gan Cao (licorice root), *Sheng Jiang* (fresh ginger rhizome), and *Da Zao* (black jujube dates) harmonize the stomach and digestive system, helping to reduce pain.

Gui Zhi (cinnamon twig) warms the body and improves circulation.

Note: This prescription should be taken with a warm cup of malted barley. Stir a tablespoon of barley malt syrup (Yi Tang) into hot water and drink with the herbal pills to improve their effectiveness.

Dosage: 8 pills three times per day.

XIAO QING LONG WAN

Minor Blue Dragon Pills
Discussion of Cold Induced Disorders
(Shang Han Lun)
Dr. Chang Chung-Ching, 142–220 A.D.

Common Usage: Common cold complicated by edema and phlegm.

Description: Early Chinese doctors noticed that there is not just one type of common cold. They realized there are several types with different symptoms which affect the body differently. In this case, an individual gets a common cold, but the body fails to resist. Fluids are retained (edema) in the chest which cause difficulty in breathing (wheezing).

A basic common cold formula will not work in a situation like this because this condition is complicated by excess phlegm and dampness. The lungs become congested with fluids without yet turning into bronchitis. The condition must still be treated as like a common cold, but with additional herbs to treat the condition correctly.

Chinese Diagnosis: An individual who already has problems retaining water or has water metabolism problems probably has underlying weak digestion and weak lungs. In this type of common cold, the lungs accumulate fluids which the Chinese call "branch drink," meaning simply that the branches of the lungs—the bronchials—are congested with fluids.

Symptoms include chills and fever without sweating, body aches, heavy head and sensitivity to cold, along with a cough, but with mucus that is clear and white, but not yellow, with bubbles perhaps. Add to these a congested, bloated chest, wheezing, and difficult urination.

Ingredients in the Formula:

Both *Ma Huang* (ephedra herb) and *Gui Zhi* (cinnamon twig) are diaphoretic (cause sweating) herbs. When a person sweats, fever is usually reduced and some congested fluids are purged. In addition, Ma Huang relaxes the bronchials and stops wheezing.

Ban Xia (pinellia rhizome) is an important herb for eliminating phlegm and helps to harmonize the middle where fluid metabolism begins.

Gan Jiang (dried ginger rhizome) warms digestion which is stifled by cold and damp from the congested fluids.

Xi Xin (asarum; wild ginger) also causes sweating and helps to stop coughing. It warms digestion and assists in clearing excess fluids which can affect the lungs and nasal passages.

Wu Wei Zi (schisandra fruit) stops coughing. *Bai Shao* (white peony root) is astringent like Wu Wei Zi; both herbs help to balance the formula to prevent excessive sweating which would damage normal body fluids.

Gan Cao (licorice root) harmonizes the formula and improves digestion.

Note: This formula should not be used long term, and it is very important that it be used to treat the right kind of cough. It would not be appropriate for use unless there is some kind of edema or water retention and the phlegm is clear or white.

Dosage: 8 pills three times per day.

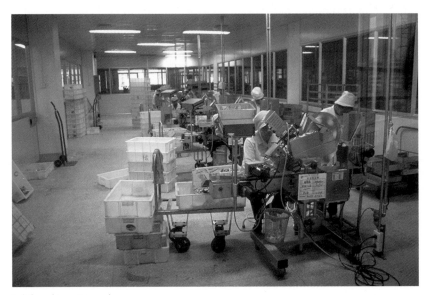

Label machines, Pangaoshou

XIN YI WAN

Magnolia Flower Pills
Formulas to Aid the Living
(Ji Sheng Fang)
Dr. Yan Yong-He, 1253 A.D.

Common Usage: Nasal congestion, stuffy nose, allergies, sinus headache.

Description: This prescription improves breathing when the nose is congested with phlegm either from common cold, allergies or other reasons. Xin Yi Wan opens the nasal passages and allows the patient to breathe more easily. It eliminates copious nasal congestion and pain from sinus headache, improving the ability to smell.

It can be taken in conjunction with other formulas to fight a common cold with chills and fever, body aches and clear mucus. It can also be taken during an allergic attack of sneezing and runny nose to alleviate symptoms.

Ingredients in the Formula:
Xin Yi Hua (magnolia flower) opens nasal passages, dries phlegm and dampness in the sinus cavities, and improves breathing.

Fang Feng (siler; ledebouriella root) guards against wind which carries pollen and other allergens, and controls the pores to protect against the invasion of wind-borne pathogens. In Chinese Medicine, all common colds are associated with wind.

Xi Xin (asarum; wild ginger) is very drying. It clears mucus from the sinuses and opens the nose to improve breathing.

Bai Zhi (angelica dahurica) dries dampness and clears the sinuses of phlegm. In Chinese Medicine, when digestion is deficient, the body accumulates fluids which congeal to become phlegm that clogs the nasal passages, bronchials and lungs.

Qiang Huo (notopterygium rhizome) and *Gao Ben* (ligusticum sinense rhizome) eliminate tension in the neck and shoulders, relieve headache pain, and direct the energy of the other herbs up to the chest, neck, and head. They are both very drying and reduce the symptoms of a common cold.

Sheng Ma (cimicifuga rhizome) directs the energy up to the head where it helps to relieve swelling and reduce heat and toxins.

Chuan Xiong (ligusticum root) eliminates sinus headache, breaks up stagnation and improves breathing.

Mu Tong (akebia stem) opens blocked water passages and drains dampness downward to clear excess phlegm which may be clogging the sinuses.

Gan Cao (licorice root) harmonizes the herbs in this formula.

Dosage: 8 pills three times per day.

XUE FU ZHU YU TANG WAN

Remove Stagnation from the Blood House Formula
Stasis in the Mansion of Blood
Corrections of Errors Among Physicians
(Yi Lin Gai Cuo)
Dr. Wang Qing-Ren, 1830 A.D.

Warning: Please see a licensed practitioner before using this product.

Common Usage: Angina or sharp pains in the chest, trauma, injury.

Description: This formula is a variation of Tao Hong Si Wu Tang (see page180). While containing almost the same basic formula, it adds other herbs to the prescription to help redirect Qi from the chest where it stagnates, causing pain. The most common usage of this formula would be when there are chronic, recurring pains in the chest from heart disease.

Chinese Diagnosis: When there is pain, there is concurrent blockage or constriction which is causing the pain. When the blockage is cleared, the pain goes away. In Chinese Medicine, angina pain is caused by heart blood stagnation. If the coronary arteries are clogged with cholesterol, blood cannot move freely through the heart to nourish the heart muscle.

Symptoms often include sharp chest pains, painful, fixed headache, heat in the chest area, insomnia, palpitations, and purple lips and tongue. These difficulties are sometimes accompanied by nausea and vomiting.

This formula includes herbs which build healthy blood as well as break up stagnation in the blood. In addition, it includes herbs to regulate the Qi which drives the blood. It also contains herbs that direct energy upward to the head and downward below the diaphragm.

Ingredients in the Formula:

Tao Hong Si Wu Tang (Peach Kernel and Safflower plus Four Substances Formula; see page 180) contains the four herbs in Si Wu Tang Wan with the substitution of *Chi Shao* (red peony root) for *Bai Shao* (white peony root) because Chi Shao more strongly moves blood. *Tao Ren* (peach kernel) and *Hong Hua* (safflower) are also added to invigorate the movement of blood. Thus, Tao Hong Si Wu Tang Wan is ideally used to remedy blood stagnation along with concurrent blood deficiency. It nourishes blood, but focuses more in this formula on invigorating blood to keep it from creating blockages.

Unique to this formula is its quality of directing Qi both up and down in the body at the same time. Two herbs direct Qi upwards while two herbs direct Qi downwards. Both help to break up stagnation by using opposing forces to balance their actions.

Chai Hu (bupleurum root) relieves liver Qi stagnation which can cause chest pain. The liver controls the free flow of Qi in the body and therefore affects the flow of blood. Chai Hu eases the stagnation of blood in the chest and directs the natural upward flow of Qi.

Zhi Ke (ripe aurantium fruit) breaks up stagnation above the diaphragm and directs energy downward away from the chest. Zhi Ke also breaks up phlegm and Qi stagnation. Arteriosclerosis (in advanced stages referred to as hardening of the arteries) can be seen in Chinese Medicine as blood and phlegm stagnation in the vessels. The coronary arteries are quite susceptible to problems of life-threatening blockages which can be reduced by this prescription.

Niu Xi (achyranthes root) directs blood downward away from the chest, breaks up blood stagnation, and nourishes the liver and the kidneys which control tendons and bones and influence the body's production of blood.

Jie Geng (platycodon root) directs energy upwards and regulates the normal functioning of the lungs which are also found above the diaphragm. When the functioning of the lungs improves, blood circulation also improves. Jie Geng promotes healthy function also by lifting the Qi derived from food up to the lungs where it can be carried to all parts of the body, thus improving nourishment of all the cells.

Gan Cao (licorice root) harmonizes the herbs in this formula.

Note: This product can also be taken after head injuries when it is certain that the bleeding has stopped. It also can be taken after any physical trauma or injury, including after delivery of a baby, again if certain that the bleeding has stopped. By breaking up blood stagnation, this formula heals bruises and injuries. Any inflammation or bruise is simply blood stagnation, blood that has escaped the vessels and capillaries. When that stagnation is broken up, an injury heals more quickly.

Dosage: 8 pills three times per day.

YAN HU SUO WAN

Great Corydalis Pills
Modern Formula

Common Usage: Stops menstrual cramps.

Description: This is a very popular patent medicine in modern China. It is used primarily by women during their menstrual cycle to stop cramping. It is most useful for difficult or painful menstruation, stopping sharp, piercing, abdominal pain and spasms. It can be taken for other similar types of discomfort, especially abdominal pain, not associated with menses.

Ingredients in the Formula:
Yan Hu Suo (corydalis rhizome) breaks up blood and Qi stagnation and alleviates chest pain, abdominal pain, menstrual pain, hernia and stomach pain.

Dosage: 8 pills three times per day.

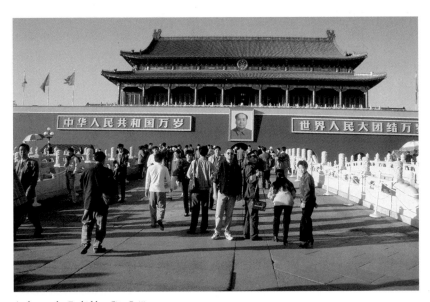

Author at the Forbidden City, Beijing

YOU GUI WAN

Restore the Right Kidney Pills
Right-Side Replenishing
Collected Treatises of Zhang Jing-Yue
(Jing Yue Quan Shu)
Dr. Zhang Jing-Yue, 1624 A.D.

Common Usage: Impotence, exhaustion, age-related problems.

Description: As a person ages, especially after the age of forty, the kidney energy begins to wane. According to some theories, the right kidney controls kidney yang energy—the fire of life energy, warmth, strength and sexual potency. In this case, You Gui Wan restores the right kidney energy or kidney yang.

Kidney yang deficiency symptoms include a sore lower back, sore knees, cold hands and feet, as well as a general overall malaise, exhaustion and poor digestion.

This is a warming formula and can be difficult for those with poor digestion. It should be taken only by those who are truly suffering from kidney yang deficiency, not by those who are simply tired or worn out.

Ingredients in the Formula:

This is a variation of *Liu Wei Di Huang Wan* (see page 85) and contains several herbs also found in Liu Wei: *Shu Di Huang* (prepared rehmannia root), *Shan Zhu Yu* (cornus fruit) and *Shan Yao* (dioscorea root). These herbs nourish the blood, elevate Qi and assist the body to retain the vital life force essence. Shu Di Huang tonifies both yin and blood. Shan Zhu Yu strengthens the kidneys and the liver which helps to support all the other organs. Shan Yao supports the kidneys and the spleen, improves digestion and lifts Qi.

Gou Qi Zi (lycium fruit) nourishes the liver and the kidneys, promotes the building of blood and yin.

Rou Gui (cinnamon bark) warms kidney fire, improves digestion and assimilation when the digestive fire is weak. It also warms cold kidneys when the life gate fire has dimmed.

Tu Si Zi (cuscuta seed) strengthens the lower back, nourishes the kidneys and tonifies both yin and yang as well as the life force essence, rebuilding a healthy foundation.

Du Zhong (eucommia bark) strengthens the liver and the kidneys and helps strengthen the lower back, knees and ankles. By helping the liver and kidneys, Du Zhong strengthens the tendons and bones.

Dang Gui (angelica sinensis) nourishes blood, expels cold, and helps reduce arthritis pain by moving blood.

Dosage: 8 pills three times per day

YU PING FENG SAN WAN

Jade Screen Powder Pills
The Teachings of Zhu Dan-Xi
(Dan Xi Xin Fa)
Dr. Zhu Dan-Xi, 1481 A.D.

Common Usage: Frequent common colds, allergies.

Description: This three-herb formula treats a deficient, weak immune system which makes an individual vulnerable to a common cold, flu, and allergies. It can be used to promote immunity to Chronic Fatigue Syndrome or Epstein-Barr.

Chinese Diagnosis: An individual who is frequently sick or suffers from allergies has a Wei Qi (defensive or protective Qi) deficiency. Wei Qi protects the body from external evils (pathogens such as bacteria, viruses, and allergens). Wei Qi is the body's first line of defense against any infectious disease. A person with weak Wei Qi more easily catches cold, more frequently catches colds, and is more susceptible to allergies, such as hay fever.

Ingredients in the Formula:
Huang Qi (astragalus root) promotes the body's overall energy, strengthening both digestion and the body's surface energy, which is controlled by the lungs. The body derives nutrients from food and then transforms that food into Qi which is carried to the lungs where it is dispersed throughout the body. In order to protect the body, the lungs send out Wei Qi to the skin layer where it provides defense from external evils. It protects the exterior of the body from wind and cold.

Bai Zhu (atractylodes rhizome) strengthens digestion. When digestion is strong, the body extracts nutrients effectively and will be better able to resist disease. This herb focuses on the need to replenish the protective energy of the body so that it does not become easily depleted. Bai Zhu also stabilizes the exterior of the body and protects the body from wind and cold.

Fang Feng (siler; ledebouriella root) guards against wind which carries pathogens and allergens such as dust, pollen and animal dander. The name

Fang Feng literally translates to "guard against wind," thus protecting the body from wind-borne disease.

Unlike Western medicine which sees allergies as an aversion to particular substances, such as an allergic reaction to dairy products or a sneezing reaction to a particular type of pollen, Chinese Medicine looks to strengthen resistance and to improve digestion as a means of combating external evils. When the body is sufficiently strong, it will not be affected by colds or the pollen season.

Note: It may take some time, perhaps as long as a month, before some effects can be seen, such as less frequent and less severe colds and perhaps as long as five months before full effects are seen. Herbal products are not like sledgehammer drugs which rely on immediate results. Herbs work slowly and heal over time to provide lasting results without nasty side effects. Unlike antihistamine drugs, herb formulas to reduce allergic reactions do not cause drowsiness and impaired motor functioning.

Dosage: 8 pills three times per day.

YU QUAN WAN

Jade Spring Pills
Modern Formula

Common Usage: Diabetes, frequent urination, stops excessive thirst.

Description: This formula alleviates some of the difficulties faced by those suffering from diabetes. It can be used by those with non-insulin dependent diabetes and can help reduce the dosage required by those who are insulin dependent.

There are two main types of diabetes: Type I diabetes is characterized by excessive urination, excessive appetite, excessive thirst, sugar in the urine and a thin body type. Type I diabetes is also called juvenile onset or insulin-dependent diabetes. Type II, or adult onset diabetes, is often associated with the excessive consumption of sweets resulting in obesity. It is related to dietary habits and lifestyle considerations. It often occurs later in life and can be controlled, in some cases, without the use of insulin.

Chinese Diagnosis: Diabetes and the symptoms of diabetes are called "Wasting and Thirsting Disorder." It is called this because people with this condition are often very thirsty and must drink a lot of water. They are often very thin and have low energy, especially those with Type I, and are seen to be "wasting away."

They also often experience a dry mouth and have a red, cracked tongue without any coating.

The above are symptoms of yin deficiency, a common diagnosis of patients in Traditional Chinese Medical Clinics. Yin deficiency heat is generated when normal levels of essential body fluids become deficient. Without those fluids, Yang heat can rise up in the body to create various problems, such as dry mouth, dry cough, hot flashes, flushed face, and other conditions. When the same body fluids are at normal levels, the Yang heat is balanced and the body is in harmony, the skin is nourished and has luster, the scalp is healthy, not dry, and the hair is thick and vital.

In Chinese Medicine, this condition can affect any or all of three organs—lungs, stomach or kidneys.

1. Lung Yin deficiency is characterized as a more mild condition leading to thirst, a dry mouth and throat and a desire to constantly drink water.
2. Stomach yin deficiency leads to excessive eating. This individual is always hungry, skinny, thirsty and often tired.
3. Kidney Yin deficiency shows up with cloudy, sugary urination, night sweats, afternoon fever, red, flushed cheeks, and lower back pain.

This formula replenishes body fluids lost from excessive urination, cools heat in the stomach, lungs and kidneys, and builds up strength and energy in a depleted individual.

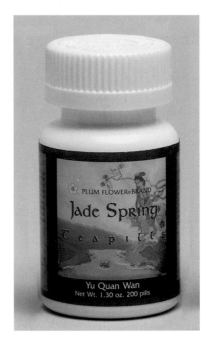

Ingredients in the Formula:
Fu Ling (poria cocos fungus) normalizes fluids in the body and strengthens digestion.

Dang Shen (codonopsis root) improves digestion and strengthens the lungs so that the body can better utilize oxygen. By improving digestion, the body can make adequate blood which in turn nourishes all the organs and the skin, carrying nutrients and vital fluids to every cell in the body. In assisting the digestive system and the lungs, it promotes normal body function and builds Qi.

Huang Qi (astragalus root) strengthens digestion, builds the immune system and helps to produce blood. For those who experience recurrent common cold, Huang Qi helps to protect against infection. It is also beneficial for the treatment of general fatigue. Huang Qi and Dang Shen together build energy, improve digestion and strengthen the lungs. Huang Qi also helps to control the pores and prevents excessive sweating.

Shu Di Huang (prepared rehmannia root) nourishes body fluids and blood. It strengthens the kidneys which are the foundation of overall good health in the body.

Ge Gen (kudzu; pueraria root) helps replenish fluids, improves thirst and cools heat in the stomach.

Wu Mei (prunus mume fruit) strengthens the lungs, stops thirst and helps to restrain the loss of vital body fluids.

Wu Wei Zi (schisandra fruit) helps prevent the loss of essential body fluids, which in diabetes are excessively excreted in the urine, by decreasing urinary frequency. It strengthens the lungs and kidneys, stops excessive sweating, and protects the heart.

Tian Hua Fen (trichosanthes kirilowii root) prevents thirst by helping to promote essential body fluids and clears heat which burns up those same fluids.

Mai Men Dong (ophiopogonis tuber) clears heat from the stomach and lungs, helps to generate fluids to cool the body, and moistens the stool to eliminate dry stool, often a symptom of those with diabetes.

Gan Cao (licorice root) harmonizes the herbs in the formula.

Dosage: 8 pills three times per day.

ZHEN WU TANG WAN

True Warrior Pills
Discussion of Cold-Induced Disorders
(Shang Han Lun)
Dr. Chang Chung-Ching, 142–220 A.D.

Special Warning: This is potentially a very serious condition. It is highly recommended that any person with the signs or symptoms listed below be taken immediately to a licensed practitioner.

Common Usage: Extreme fatigue and sleepiness.

Description: Strengthens the debilitated, and warms the interior.

Symptoms include excessive sweating, difficult urination, edema, heavy head, cold hands and feet, fatigue, shaking and sleepiness.

Note: This is an extreme type of fatigue and the above formula should not be taken by anyone who shows any kind of heat signs.

Chinese Diagnosis: Zhen Wu Tang was originally formulated by Dr. Chang as a treatment for the common cold, but specifically a wind-cold common cold when the Yang Qi was injured and the spleen Qi was very weak with symptoms of dampness, fatigue, shaking and sleepiness.

Ingredients in the Formula:

Dang Shen (codonopsis root) builds energy and improves digestion. It strengthens the function of the lungs and the immune system.

Bai Zhu (atractylodes rhizome) dries dampness and improves digestion, thus building the immune system and lifting Qi.

Bai Shao (white peony root) builds blood and helps improve the protective (Wei) Qi. It also helps to stop muscle spasms along with Gan Cao (see below) and balances the warming properties of the other herbs in the formula.

Fang Feng (siler; ledebouriella root) guards against wind by protecting the skin layer and eliminates shaking and twitching.

Rou Gui (cinnamon bark) and *Gan Jiang* (dried ginger rhizome) warm the interior (the internal core) and strengthen the kidneys and digestion. They help reduce arthritis pain and improve mobility in stiff joints.

Gan Cao (licorice root) harmonizes the formula and improves energy.

Dosage: 8 pills three times per day.

ZUO GUI WAN

Restore the Left Kidney Pills
Left-Side Replenishing Pills
Collected Treatises of Zhang Jing-Yue
(Jing Yue Quan Shu)
Dr. Zhang Jing-Yue, 1624 A.D.

Common Usage: Fortifies kidney function.

Description: A companion of You Gui Wan (Right-Side Replenishing Pills; see page 200), this formula treats lower back pain but from a different cause, that of depleted vital life force essence. The symptoms include heat conditions, such as night sweats, dry mouth, thirst with a desire to drink cold fluids, as well as weak legs, dizziness, ear ringing and blurry vision.

Note: This formula is harder to digest than Liu Wei Di Huang Wan (Six Flavor Tea Pills; see page 85) and therefore must be taken carefully by those with poor digestion.

Ingredients in the Formula:

This prescription contains three herbs from Liu Wei: *Shu Di Huang* (prepared rehmannia root), *Shan Yao* (dioscorea root), and *Shan Zhu Yu* (cornus fruit) which build blood, elevate Qi and help to retain the vital life force essence. Together, they build vital fluids and blood by improving digestion.

Gou Qi Zi (lycium fruit) nourishes liver blood and strengthens the kidneys which support all the other organs in the body.

Niu Xi (achyranthes root) directs energy downward in the body to the root and source of vitality, assists the liver and kidneys, plus it strengthens the lower back and tendons.

Tu Si Zi (cuscuta seed) assists kidney Yang, tonifies Yin, and strengthens the lower back (the realm of the kidneys).

Dosage: 8 pills three times per day.

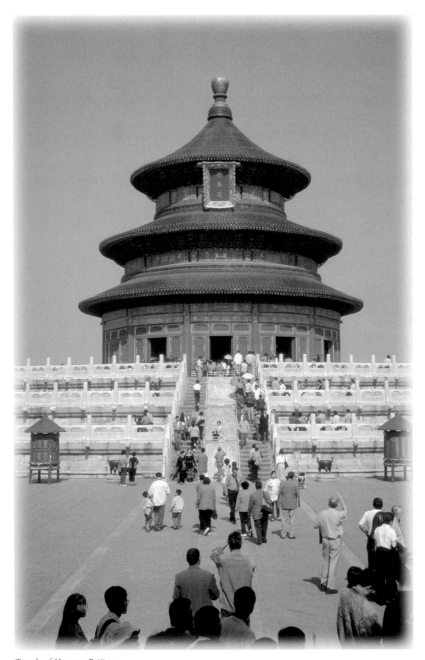

Temple of Heaven, Beijing

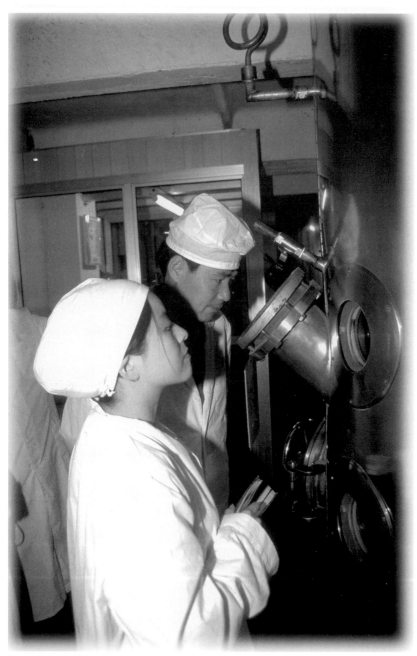

Tianjin Great Wall Brand Factory

7

OTHER HIGH-QUALITY CHINESE PRODUCTS

In this book, I feel comfortable only recommending products from companies and factories that I have personally visited. There are other companies in China which produce fine quality medicines, but unless I have personally seen the production facilities, I am reluctant to promote them. The products that I have discussed earlier in this book are manufactured under the highest quality standards and are to my knowledge among the best available. I hope in the future to visit more factories and to expand my knowledge of the production of Chinese patent remedies. Until then, the companies discussed in this book are the best that I have seen.

Originally, I hadn't planned to include these products in this book, but after seeing their production facilities and verifying the quality of their products, I felt that I had to include them. Consequently, I have not gone into as much detail with the medicines mentioned below as with those that I have discussed earlier.

PANGAOSHOU HERBAL PRODUCTS COMPANY

Certified GMP by the Australian Therapeutic Goods Administration in late 1996 (see Appendix), the Pangaoshou Herbal Products Company of Guangzhou, China, produces high-quality products in liquid form. As you will see in the accompanying photographs, this factory is meticulously maintained and extremely sanitary. I toured it soon after it opened for production in 1996 and left impressed by their excellent manufacturing facilities.

Pangaoshou Herbal Products company produces a number of products including the following:

SHOU WU TONIC ESSENCE

He Shou Wu Liquid Extract
Modern Formula

Common Usage: Restores normal hair color, builds blood.

Description: A formula to tonify blood, it is often taken to replenish sexual energy as well as to restore natural hair color. The main herb in the formula is *He Shou Wu* (polygonum multiflorum root) which means in Chinese "Black Hair Mr. He." The remaining herbs in the formula support the liver and kidneys, which control the growth and color of the hair. It must be taken for several months in order to restore normal hair color. In addition, the formula strengthens the knees and lower back, supports the softening of tendons and strengthens the function of the kidneys which support all the organs of the body.

Dosage: 1 tablespoon three times per day.

FRITILLARIA AND LOQUAT COUGH SYRUP

Modern Formula

Common Usage: Cough.

Description: As its name indicates, this product is a cough syrup. The herbs in the formula nourish and strengthen the function of the lungs and help to loosen sticky phlegm. It frees sticky phlegm so that it can be coughed up and no longer impede normal lung function. This syrup can be used both for chronic and acute cough as well as in cases of emphysema, asthma and difficult breathing.

Dosage: 1 to 3 teaspoons three to four times per day.

LOQUAT FLAVORED JELLY

Modern Formula

Common Usage: Expectorant, stops cough.

Description: Similar to the Fritillaria and Loquat Cough Syrup, the Loquat Flavored Jelly strengthens normal lung function and can help eliminate sticky phlegm that causes cough. It too can be taken to help eliminate long-term chronic cough.

Dosage: 1 to 3 teaspoons three to four times per day.

SAN SHE DAN CHUAN BEI YE

Three Snake Gallbladder and Fritillaria Liquid
Modern Formula

Common Usage: Bronchitis, cough.

Description: This product clears phlegm and heat from the lungs. It is especially useful for children who are suffering from common cold that invades the lungs and causes thick yellow phlegm. It comes in small glass vials and is effective in dealing with knotted phlegm or phlegm that is difficult to expectorate.

Dosage: 1 to 2 vials per day.

TANG KWEI GIN

Dang Gui Nourish Blood Syrup
Based on: Ba Zhen Wan
Eight Treasure Pills
Catalogued Essentials for Correcting the Body
(Zheng Ti Lei Yao)
Dr. Bi Li-Zhai, 1529 A.D.

Common Usage: Anemia, blood deficiency.

Description: As its title indicates, this formula is designed to help replenish blood, lost as a result of either accident, trauma, injury or poor digestion. It will also benefit women who lose blood every month with menstruation and who don't replace it well. See Ba Zhen Wan, page 55.

There is a red box version of this formula which is widely available that contains sugar. The formula from the Pangaoshou Factory contains no sugar, drugs or alcohol.

Dosage: 1 tablespoon two times per day.

TIANJIN GREAT WALL BRAND PRODUCTS

I visited three facilities in Tianjin during October 1996 and found them to be excellent. One of the factories operated by this company was certified GMP almost 10 years ago, and even though it has been operating for years, it is still in GMP condition. This company has a good reputation and its products can be found in most Chinese herb shops in China and the U.S. They also manufacture products for the Japanese who prefer freeze-dried powders to pills which are more popular in the U.S. My teachers at the clinic where I was a student consider Tianjin products to be of the highest quality and claim that they get excellent results when using them. My own experience with my patients has verified their effectiveness, so I am happy to recommend them.

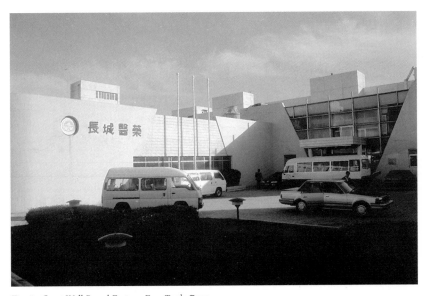

Tianjin Great Wall Brand Factory, Free Trade Zone

YIN QIAO JIE DU PIAN

Honeysuckle and Forsythia Clear Toxins Pills
Systematic Differentiation of Warm Diseases
(Wen Bing Tiao Bian)
Dr. Wu Ju-Tong, 1798 A.D.

Warning: Beware of counterfeit versions of this product. I have seen several different counterfeits because this formula is so popular. There are many legitimate manufacturers of Yin Qiao, but I have not visited the factories and cannot therefore vouch for the quality of production.

Common Usage: Common cold with sore throat and fever. (See page 121 for a complete discussion of this formula.)

Description: There are two variations of this product: one comes with sugar coated pills (some versions contain synthetic drugs); the other in small glass vials of 8 uncoated pills each. Both are very good, but I prefer the uncoated product.

Look for a Plum Flower version of these products to ensure that you are getting good quality. I have seen so many different types of packaging and products that it is very difficult to determine which is legitimate and of good quality. Therefore, I always buy Plum Flower Brand because I know it is good quality.

Dosage: 4 pills three times per day.

CHIN KOO TIEH SHANG WAN

Jin Gu Die Shang Wan
Muscle and Bone Trauma Injury Pills
Modern Formula

Common Usage: Heals bruises, sprains, strains, contusions, fractures, and other traumatic injuries. See page 168 for a complete discussion of this product. It is also available from Plum Flower.

Dosage: 10 pills two to three times per day.

CHIEN CHIN CHIH TAI WAN

Thousand Pieces of Gold Stop Leukorrhea Pills
Modern Formula
[Based on: Gu Jing Wan]
Stabilize the Menses Pills
Introduction to Medicine
Yi Xue Ru Me
Dr. Li Ting, 1575 A.D.

Common Usage: Vaginal discharge.

Description: Like Yu Dai Wan, this formula is useful in treating vaginal discharge. Although there are at least two major causes of leukorrhea, this formula addresses both types: a spleen Qi deficiency type and a lower burner, damp heat type. In the case of lower burner damp heat, the dampness stagnates and accumulates below the navel where it restricts the normal flow of fluids and Qi. Whenever there is a stagnation of dampness, it will eventually turn into heat. Where there is an accumulation of dampness, it will eventually overflow. In this situation, the excess fluids are forced out in the form of vaginal discharge.

This is also the case with spleen Qi deficiency discharge. The spleen is responsible for the proper movement and transportation of fluids in the body. When the spleen is deficient, fluids can stagnate in the lower burner which includes the kidneys, bladder and uterus. In this scenario, the fluids overflow and leak out through the vagina.

See Yu Dai Wan, page 123. There may be a Plum Flower version of this product available soon.

Dosage: 10 pills one time per day.

CHING FEI YI HUO PIAN

Clear Lung Heat Pills
Modern Formula
Based on: Qing Qi Hua Tan Wan
Clear Qi Transform Phlegm Pills
Investigations of Medical Formulas
(Yi Fang Kao)
Dr. Wu Kun, 1584 A.D.

Caution: This product should not be used during pregnancy. Not to be taken long-term. Discontinue usage after heat signs diminish.

Common Usage: Phlegm congestion in lungs.

Description: I have used this formula many times with my patients with positive results. It can be used for any type of lung infection with yellow phlegm. Very often when someone gets a common cold, the infection moves internally into the lungs and causes congestion, cough and wheezing. This formula can be used to treat most types of lung heat conditions with cough, sore throat and residual fever that remains following a common cold. It should not be used long term for any type of chronic cough or lung condition.

See Qing Qi Hua Tan Wan, page 96. Look for the Plum Flower version of this product to ensure that you are not buying a counterfeit.

Dosage: 4 pills two to three times per day.

HUANG LIAN SHANG CHING PIAN

Coptis Upper Burner Heat Clearing Pills
[Based on: Huang Lian Jie Du Tang]
Arcane Essentials from the Imperial Library
(Wai Tai Bi Yao)
Dr. Wang Tao, 752 A.D.

Caution: Do not use during pregnancy. Nor should it be used long-term. If you experience diarrhea, discontinue.

Common Usage: Tonsillitis, mouth sores, bronchitis, ear infections.

Description: This formula is excellent for any type of infection in the upper body such as ear infections, tonsillitis, red eyes, mouth sores, and sore gums. I have often recommended this product to my patients for swollen glands and ear infections with good results.

It is also beneficial for any type of hot, inflamed skin problem, such as skin rash, poison oak, hives, carbuncles, and boils.

Look for a Plum Flower version of this product.

Dosage: 4 pills one to two times per day.

LIEN CHIAO PAI DU PIAN

Forsythia Clear Toxins Pills
Modern Formula

Caution: Do not use during pregnancy.

Common Usage: Skin infections.

Description: This formula is intended for any type of skin infection and red swollen skin problem such as hives or poison oak. It can be used for boils, carbuncles, and skin infections with pus, any skin problem with red, itching skin. It can also be used with fever and illnesses accompanying skin conditions.

Look for a Plum Flower version of this product.

Dosage: 2 to 4 pills two to three times per day.

NIU HUANG CHIEH TU PIAN

Bezoar Clear Toxins Pills
Modern Formula

Caution: It should not be used during pregnancy. Not recommended for long-term use.

Description: An excellent product for children's ear infections, ear ache, red eyes, toothache, sore throat and mouth sores.

Dosage: 4 pills two times per day.

GUANGZHOU QI XING FACTORY

This is another excellent facility, being certified GMP in late 1996 by the Australian Therapeutic Goods Administration. (See Appendix, p. 268.) I visited this factory in both October 1996 and October 1997, but was not allowed to take photographs inside the manufacturing facility. I can, however, attest that the production quality, cleanliness and machinery compare favorably with the best facilities that I have seen. This is a relatively new factory and they were constructing new production facilities during our first visit.

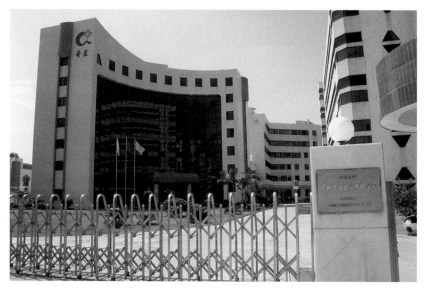

Guangzhou Qi Xing Factory

GAN MAO LING

Common Cold Effective Remedy
Modern Formula
Plum Flower Brand

Caution: Plum Flower Gan Mao Ling is the only brand that I can recommend. Other versions have been tested and have been found to contain pharmaceutical drugs and synthetic dyes. I have seen many different variations of this product over the years, most of which were probably smuggled into the U.S. Some versions of this formula are of questionable quality and may be counterfeit.

Common Usage: Common cold.

Description: This is the most popular and effective Chinese common cold pill available in the U.S. because it treats both colds and flu. It will treat any type of common cold—wind-cold and wind-heat. Also, it is quite popular because it is not necessary to distinguish between wind-cold or wind-heat before using it.

As with any treatment of common cold, it should be taken at the first sign of symptoms in order to be effective. It is advisable when coming down with a cold or flu to stay warm and to encourage sweating.

Symptoms include sudden, unexplained fatigue, chills and fever, sore throat, body aches, neck aches and swollen glands.

Dosage: 4 or 5 pills three times per day.

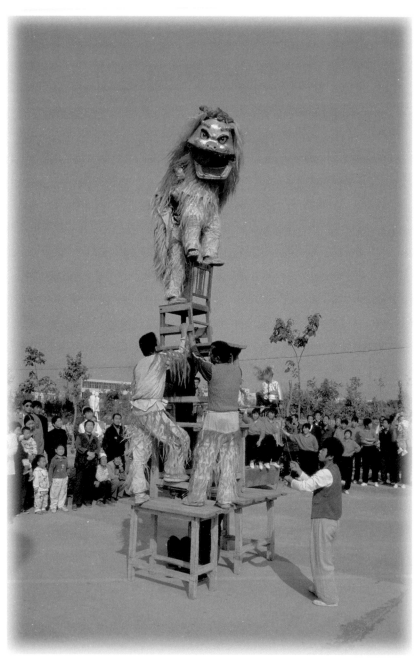

Dragon Dance, Opening Ceremonies, Mayway Anguo

8

OTHER CHINESE
PATENT MEDICINES

The following products are very popular in Chinese herb shops here in the U.S. as well as in foreign countries. Many of these products are untested, however, and may be compromised with pharmaceutical drugs, heavy metals and synthetic dyes. When I know that a product has been tested, or I am aware of products which are high-quality alternatives, I will mention it in this text. This is very important because many of these products, though effective and popular, are unfortunately of unknown quality.

Several books have been written that describe the uses of Chinese herb formulas in pill form, but none of the books addresses the issues of quality control, contamination and counterfeiting. Unfortunately, many popular products may be compromised without the author's knowledge.

I have also included some products manufactured by American companies which I have seen in Health Food stores. Most of the products produced by American companies are based on Classic Chinese formulas, such as Yin Qiao Jie Du Pien (see pages 121, 214), so I haven't listed them in this section.

AN MIEN PIAN

Peaceful Sleep Pills
[Based on: Suan Zao Ren Tang]
Essentials from the Golden Cabinet
(Jin Gue Yao Lue)
Dr. Chang Chung-Ching, 142–220 A.D.
China National Native Products, Hopei

Common Usage: Insomnia.

Description: This formula is very popular in herb stores in China as well as in the U.S. It cools liver heat, reduces stress, and calms the mind, encouraging sleep. Symptoms can include anxiety, restlessness, red eyes, poor memory and mental weariness.

I have not visited this factory and cannot verify the quality of this product, but it has been tested and does not contain any drugs. It probably contains synthetic red dye.

There is a Plum Flower Brand version of this that is now available.

Dosage: 4 pills three times per day.

ARMADILLO COUNTER POISON PILLS

Chuan Shan Jia Chu Shi Ching Du Wan
Modern Formula
United Pharmaceutical Works, Guangdong Province

Common Usage: Skin itching, rash, poison oak.

Description: This is a very effective product to stop skin itching, either from rash, poison oak or other causes. It can be used for any type of skin condition in which the skin is red, inflamed and itching.

I have not visited this factory and the pills may contain synthetic red dye. As far as I know, it has not been tested for drugs.

Dosage: 5 pills three times per day.

ASTRA 8

Eight Herbs with Astragalus
Modern Formula
Health Concerns

Common Usage: Boosts immune system.

Description: This formula is especially valuable in building the immune system. I highly recommend it, even though it is not produced according to the standards of the best factories in China. It is made of herb extracts or herb powders which are blended together and then pressed into tablets here in the U.S.

I have visited Health Concerns' manufacturing facilities and have found the conditions there to be of good quality. This product has not been tested, but I have been assured by the manufacturer that it is free of chemicals and synthetic colors.

ASTRAGALUS 10

Ten Herbs with Astragalus
Modern Formula
Seven Forests

Common Usage: Boosts immune system.

Description: See Astra 8 above. These are very similar formulas to strengthen the immune system and to eliminate chronic illness.

I have visited the manufacturing facilities and found them to be satisfactory. This product has not been tested, but probably does not contain drugs or food coloring.

BAO JI WAN

Po Chai Pills
Modern Formula
Li Chung Shing Tong Factory, Hong Kong

Common Usage: Stomach upset.

Description: This is virtually identical to Pill Curing (see below); it has almost the same ingredients and contains synthetic red dye. As far as I know it has not been tested.

Dosage: 1 to 3 vials per time; can be taken three to four times per day as necessary.

BI YAN PIAN

Nose Inflammation Pills
[Based on: Cang Er Zi San]
Xanthium Powder
Formulas to Aid the Living
(Ji Sheng Fan)
Dr. Yan Yong-He, 1253 A.D.
Chung Lien Drug Works, Wuchang, Hubei Province

Common Usage: Allergies, nasal congestion.

Description: Bi Yan Pian dries mucus and helps to open nasal passages. It contains herbs which dry dampness and phlegm, fight nasal infections and kill pathogenic bacteria. It can also be taken along with cold formulas such as Gan Mao Ling (see page 219) and Yin Qiao Jie Du Pian (see page 121) to fight colds and to clear a stuffy nose.

Laboratory tests show that it contains acetaminophen (Tylenol) and it probably also contains synthetic dye.

Plum Flower Brand Bi Yan Pian is currently available and does not contain dyes or pharmaceutical drugs.

Dosage: 3 to 4 tablets three times per day.

BUTIAO TABLETS

Nourish Blood Regulate Menses Pills
Modern Formula
United Pharmaceutical Manufactory, Guangzhou

Common Usage: Regulates the menses.

Description: This formula builds blood, regulates the menstrual cycle and harmonizes a woman's body. It supports the kidneys, regulates the liver which controls the flow of blood, and warms the internal organs. It helps alleviate cramps, insomnia, headaches associated with menses, moodiness and irregular cycles.

I have not visited this factory and therefore cannot address issues of quality of production. It has not been tested.

Dosage: 3 pills two to three times a day as needed.

CEREBRAL TONIC PILLS

Bu Nao Wan
Modern Formula
Xian Chinese Pharmaceutical Works, Xian, Shaanxi Province

Common Usage: Calms the mind.

Description: This formula works to soothe the mind and relax the heart. It has an overall calming effect, reducing anxiety, improving memory, and sleep. It can also alleviate other mental problems, such as neurasthenia, panic attacks and phobias.

I have not visited this factory and therefore cannot address issues of quality of production or purity. It has not been tested.

Dosage: 10 pills three times per day.

CHI KUAN YEN WAN

Bronchitis, Cough, Phlegm, Difficult Breathing Pills
Modern Formula
Dr. Shih Chin-Mo
Beijing Tung Jen Tang, Beijing

Common Usage: Cough, bronchitis.

Description: As indicated by the title, this is a formula for bronchitis, cough, phlegm and difficult breathing brought on by a common cold that has invaded the chest and lungs.

I have not visited this factory and therefore cannot address issues of quality of production or purity. It has not been tested for drugs, but I suspect that it contains synthetic colors.

Dosage: 20 pills two times per day.

CHIEN CHIN CHIH TAI WAN

Woman Stop Leukorrhea Pills
Compendium of Therapy for Women's Diseases
(Ji Yin Gang Mu)
Author Unknown, Qing Dynasty, 1644–1911 A.D.
Tianjin Drug Manufactory, Tianjin, Hebei Province

Caution: Beware of counterfeits of this product.

Common Usage: Leukorrhea, vaginal discharge.

Description: Like Yu Dai Wan, this product is intended to stop vaginal discharge, especially from deficiency of blood and Qi. It basically means that a woman's body is not strong enough to control the fluids in her body, allowing them to leak out the vagina. It is primarily a digestive problem, because in Chinese Medicine the digestion controls and disperses body fluids to their proper locations. When this mechanism fails, fluids accumulate in areas where they don't belong and the body tries to purge them.

The Tianjin factory is very high quality. I visited three of their facilities in October 1996 and was favorably impressed by their production methods. I can highly recommend this product. It contains no drugs or synthetic dyes.

Dosage: 10 pills once a day.

CHING CHUN BAO

Green Vitality Pills
Modern Formula
Hangzhou Medicine Factory #2, Hangzhou, Zhejian Province

Common Usage: Improves energy

Description: This prescription is very popular in China. It strengthens the kidneys and sexual energy, reduces fatigue, and slows the aging process. It also improves memory, builds the immune system, and guards against sickness.

I have not visited this factory and therefore cannot address issues of quality of production or purity. It has not been tested.

Dosage: 2 pills two times a day or as needed.

CHING FEI YI HUO PIAN

Clear Lung Eliminate Fire Pills
Modern Formula
Tianjin Drug Manufactory, Tianjin, Hebei Province

Caution: Unfortunately, there are many counterfeits of this product. I do not have an example of counterfeit packaging at this time. There is a Plum Flower version which contains no synthetic drugs or artificial colors.

Common Usage: Lung infection, bronchitis with yellow phlegm.

Description: An excellent formula for clearing heat and phlegm from the lungs. It can be used like an antibiotic to fight lung infections such as bronchitis and can also be used in the aftermath of illness to clear up residual lung heat and sticky phlegm.

I recommend this product because it is very high quality. I have visited the factory and observed the manufacturing, which I found to be of the highest level. Doctors who I greatly respect tell me that products produced by this factory are the very best in China. It has not been tested, but I am certain that it does not contain drugs, nor does it contain any synthetic colors.

Look for a Plum Flower Brand version of this product.

Dosage: 4 pills two times per day.

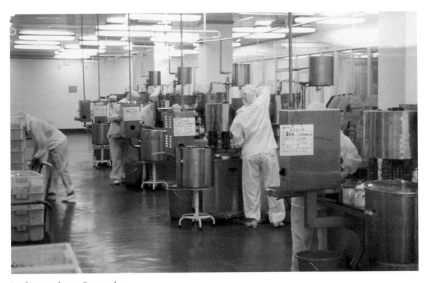

Bottling machines, Pangaoshou

CHUAN XIN LIAN

Antiphlogistic Pills
Andrographitis Herb Pills
Modern Formula
United Pharmaceutical Manufactory, Guangzhou

Common Usage: Sore throat, tonsillitis, ear infection, bladder infection.

Description: This formula is very popular with women who get bladder infections, especially those who get them repeatedly. I often recommend this to my patients along with Ba Zheng San (see page 135) because they work very well together to eliminate urinary tract infections without side effects. It works as a natural antibiotic for the treatment of any number of other problems, such as sore throat, swollen tonsils and swollen lymph glands. It can be used for both bacterial and viral infections.

This product has not yet been tested, but it probably contains synthetic dye as a tablet coloring. I have not visited this factory and therefore cannot verify the quality of production.

Plum Flower Brand Chuan Xin Lian is currently available.

Dosage: 2 to 3 pills three times per day.

COMPOUND CORTEX EUCOMMIA TABLETS

Du Zhong Pian
Modern Formula
Kweichow United Pharmaceutical Manufactory, Guizhou

Common Usage: Lowers blood pressure.

Description: This product contains four herbs, all of which have been proven in laboratory studies to reduce blood pressure in animals. In Chinese Medicine, high blood pressure is often caused by liver heat which causes liver yang to rise, elevating blood pressure. It is very common for men with high blood pressure to have red faces, red noses, red ears, red shoulders and red necks. This is a manifestation of the heat rising in the body. This formula clears liver heat and tonifies the liver and the kidneys to nourish fluids and clear heat.

I have not visited this factory, nor have I seen any tests to determine if this product contains drugs. It probably contains synthetic dyes. I have not come across any counterfeits of this product.

Dosage: 5 pills three times per day.

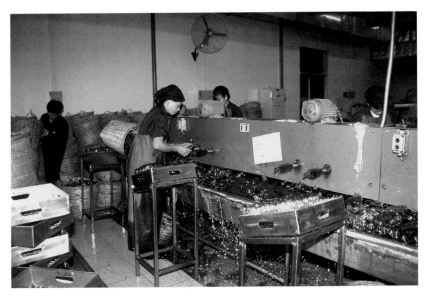

Sterilizing bottles, Pangaoshou

CORYDALIS YAN HU SUO PIAN

Corydalis Stop Pain Pills
Modern Formula
China National Pharmaceutical Corporation

Common Usage: Menstrual cramps.

Description: Yan Hu Suo reduces abdominal pain. It works as an analgesic to stop cramps both before and during menses. Some versions of this product also contain Bai Zhi and can help stop headache as well as menstrual cramps.

There are many versions of this product, but only Plum Flower Brand (see page 199) has been tested and is certain to be free of drugs and synthetic dyes.

Dosage: For pain take 1 to 2 pills three times per day.

CURING PILLS (PILL CURING)

Kan Ning Wan
Healthy Peaceful Pills
Modern Formula
Various Manufacturers

Special Warning: This product is extremely popular in China and in the U.S. There are many counterfeit versions of it. As of this writing, I don't know which is the legitimate manufacturer (See photos page 37). Most of these products probably contain synthetic red dye.

Common Usage: Stomach upset.

Description: This is easily one of the most popular products in China. It relieves almost any type of simple stomach discomfort. It can be taken after overeating or for bloating from weak digestion and can be used for any general stomach upset, nausea, gas or indigestion. It is a wonderful product and extremely helpful, especially after you have overeaten or after meals when food sits in your stomach and won't digest. It can also be taken to relieve minor food poisoning

Plum Flower has a high-quality version of Curing Pills which is manufactured in an internationally certified GMP factory. It has been tested and contains no drugs or synthetic, artificial colors.

Dosage: One to three vials at a time to resolve complications, three or four times a day as needed.

DAN SHEN PILLS

Fu Fang Dan Shen Pian
Medicinal Substance Salvia Pills
Modern Formula
Shanghai Chinese Medicine Works, Shanghai

Warning: Caution is advised when there is pain radiating down the left arm, along with heart palpitations and chest pain (angina). See a doctor immediately.

Common Usage: Regulates the heart, stops chest pain.

Description: Stops heart pain and encourages the circulation of heart blood. Dan Shen has the capability of increasing the circulation of blood through the heart by opening blood vessels to allow more blood to flow through those vessels. This is especially important in the coronary arteries.

It has not been tested for drugs. I have not visited the factory so I cannot address issues of quality. It probably contains synthetic dyes.

Plum Flower has a variation of this formula: Dan Shen Yin Wan, see page 147.

Dosage: 2 pills two times per day.

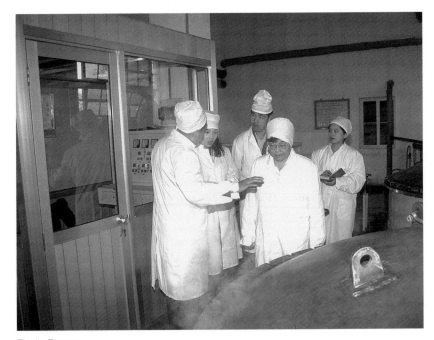

Tianjin Factory

ER XIAN TANG WAN

Two Immortals
TCM Medical Formulas from the Shuguang Hospital
of the Shanghai College of TCM
(Fang Ji Xue)
Shen's Herbal Formulas
Health Concerns

Common Usage: Menopausal symptoms.

Description: In Chinese Medicine, this prescription treats an internal condition which is called Yin and Yang not balanced. When Yin and Yang are not balanced, the body sends mixed messages, such as sweating and hot flashes accompanied by cold hands and feet. Symptoms can include sweating for no apparent reason, muscle cramps and shaking. This formula treats menopause, high blood pressure, and mental disturbances associated with aging.

I have visited the factory that does the tableting of these pills, and found the conditions to be acceptable. Two Immortals has not been tested, but probably does not contain drugs or dyes.

Dosage: 3 to 6 pills three times per day.

FARGELIN FOR PILES

Qiang Li Hua Zhi Ling
High Strength Dissipate Hemorrhoids Effective Cure
United Pharmaceutical Manufactory, Guangzhou, China
[Based on: Huai Hua San]
Formulas of Universal Benefit from My Practice
(Pu Ji Ben Shi Fang)
Dr. Xu Shu-Wei, 1132 A.D.

Common Usage: Hemorrhoids.

Description: This is a very popular formula for treating hemorrhoids and comes in two forms—regular strength and high strength.

Neither one has been tested for drugs, and both probably contain synthetic colors. I have not visited this factory.

Dosage: 4 to 6 pills three times per day.

GAN MAO TUI RE CHONG JI

Common Cold Reduce Fever Granules
Modern Formula
Various Manufacturers

Common Usage: Common cold.

Description: This is a very popular common cold formula because it can be taken like tea. It is used by tearing open a packet of crystals and dissolving them in hot water. It is good for children with a fever who cannot take pills. Similar to Gan Mao Ling.

There are many different manufacturers. I have only visited one company that produces this product—Tianjin Great Wall Brand—for which I have a great deal of respect. It has not been tested. I do not know if it contains drugs or artificial colors.

Dosage: For adults, 1 to 2 packets three times per day; for children, 1 packet two to three times a day depending on the child's body weight. A fifty-pound child should get no more than $1/_3$ the adult dose.

GE JIE DA BU WAN

Gecko Big Tonifying Pills
Modern Formula
Yulin Drug Manufactory, Guangxi Province

Common Usage: Weakness, fatigue.

Description: As suggested by the name of this formula, it is a strong tonic ideal for those who are very deficient with weakness in the liver, kidneys, and digestion. It contains gecko lizard as one of the main ingredients to reduce wheezing and asthma. It is designed for those who are weak and suffer shortness of breath, dizziness, fatigue, ear ringing, weak lower back, cold hands and feet, and poor appetite.

It has not been tested for either drugs or synthetic dyes. I have not visited the factory.

Dosage: 3 to 5 caps two times per day.

GOOD SLEEPING AND WORRY-FREE TEA PILLS

Shui De An

Modern Formula

Common Usage: Insomnia.

Description: A very popular formula for treating insomnia and for alleviating stress.

It has not been tested, and I have not visited the factory. The capsules may contain synthetic dyes.

Dosage: 2 pills three times a day or as needed.

HAWTHORN FAT-REDUCING PILLS

Jiang Ya Ping Pian

Modern Formula

Sanming Pharmaceutical Factory, Fujian

Common Usage: Lowers blood cholesterol.

Description: I have seen positive results with this product. It has dramatically and quickly reduced cholesterol in patients at the clinic where I worked.

I have not visited this factory and cannot address its quality of production. It probably contains artificial food coloring, and it has been tested for drugs, but none were detected.

Dosage: 2 to 3 pills two times per day.

HSIAO KEH CHUAN

Eliminate Cough and Asthma
Special Medicine for Bronchitis
Modern Formula
Harbin Drug Manufactory, Harbin

Common Usage: Bronchitis.

Description: This product contains only one herb, Man San Hung (Folium Rhododendri Daurici), and is not found in most herb books. It clears phlegm and heat from the lungs, and it treats bronchitis, both chronic and acute. It is both antitussive (stops cough) and helps expectorate phlegm.

The packaging of this product has been recently changed to eliminate the words "Special Medicine for Bronchitis" which had been prominent on the label. It has not been tested for drugs or synthetic dyes.

Available in both pill form and in liquid.

Dosage: Liquid: 1 tablespoon three times per day; capsules: 2 capsules three times per day.

HUANG LIAN SU PIAN

Coptis Concentrate Pills
Modern Formula
Min-Kang Drug Manufactory, Yi-Chang

Common Usage: Food poisoning, diarrhea.

Description: This is the treatment of choice for diarrhea in China. It can treat almost any type of acute diarrhea caused by food-borne or water-borne bacteria. See page 165. I have recommended this product many times to my patients with very good results, and I have used it myself on several occasions after getting sick while traveling. I recommend using it along with Mu Xiang Shun Qi Wan (see page 93) to regulate digestion and the intestines after experiencing diarrhea.

I have seen counterfeit versions of this product. It has not been tested for drugs or synthetic dyes.

Dosage: 2 to 4 pills three times per day as needed. Take three doses as a minimum before stopping use.

JI GU CAO WAN

Herba Abri Pills
Modern Formula
Yulin Drug Manufactory, Guangxi

Special Warning: The diseases listed below are potentially life-threatening. Do not attempt self-medication. Please see a licensed practitioner.

Common Usage: Hepatitis, jaundice.

Description: This formula specifically treats the liver and gallbladder and is especially useful in treating diseases such as hepatitis, jaundice and cholecystitis (gallbladder inflammation). It can also be taken as a preventative for those who feel that they may have been exposed to hepatitis.

It has not been tested for drugs or dyes. I have not visited this factory.

Dosage: 4 pills three times per day.

KAI KIT WAN

Reduce Prostate Swelling Pills
Modern Formula
Hanyang Pharmaceutical Works, Hanyang, Hubei

Common Usage: Prostate enlargement, benign prostate hypertrophy.

Description: Reduces swelling and strengthens the function of the kidneys which control the prostate. It reduces pain, drains excessive dampness and opens the orifices so that urination is easier. Enlarged prostate is fairly common in men over the age of 50 who often have difficulty urinating, especially at night. The prostate enlarges and cuts off the flow of urine through the urethra. Many men suffer from this problem and have to wake several times a night to relieve themselves. Kai Kit Wan reduces the swelling of the prostate, easing urination.

This product has not been tested and may contain synthetic colors. I have not visited this factory.

Dosage: 3 to 6 pills three times per day.

KAI YEUNG PILLS

Hua She Jie Yang Wan
Colorful Snake Anti-Itching Pills
Modern Formula
United Pharmaceutical Works, Guangzhou

Common Usage: Skin itching, rashes, poison oak.

Description: Used to treat itching skin, especially chronic skin itching. It is intended for those who are deficient, perhaps a little anemic. When blood is properly abundant, the skin is adequately nourished, and chronic skin problems often improve.

I have not visited this factory, and this product has not been tested.

Dosage: 5 pills three times per day.

KANG GU ZENG SHENG PIAN

Prevent Bone Hyperplasia Pills
Modern Formula
United Pharmaceutical Manufactory, Foshan, Guangdong Province

Common Usage: Arthritis.

Description: This treats a type of arthritis in which both the small and large joints are sore and stiff. It can help restore dislocated discs, eliminate pain from dull, achy joints, and strengthen tendons and bones to support the joints more effectively. It can be taken long term to strengthen the body's resistance to arthritis.

There may be counterfeits of this product. I have seen three versions of it (See photos on page 40). It has been tested and contains no drugs, but it probably contains synthetic dyes. I have not visited this factory.

Dosage: 6 pills three times per day.

LI DAN WAN

Benefit Gallbladder Pills
Modern Formula
Qingdao Medicine Works, Shangdong Province

Common Usage: Gallbladder problems.

Description: This is a good product to remedy gallbladder problems which are rampant in this society. The gallbladder is affected by stress and by damp heat which causes bile (which is stored in the gallbladder) to congeal, first forming a sandy substance and finally stones. In China it is said that middle-aged women over the age of forty are especially susceptible to gallbladder difficulties. In the clinic, we look for four conditions: over-weight, over forty, fertile and female. Gallbladder problems are not limited to women. Men are also affected. Some symptoms are right shoulder pain, pain at the lower border of the right ribs, waking between 11 P.M. and 1 A.M., difficulty digesting fats and the need to evacuate your bowels immediately after eating.

This product has not been tested for drugs and probably contains synthetic dyes. I have not visited this factory.

Dosage: 5 pills three times per day.

LI FEI TANG YI PIAN

Benefit Lungs Pills
Pulmonary Tonic Pills
China National Native Produce & Animal Import
and Export Corporation, Hebei, China

Common Usage: Weak lungs, shortness of breath, chronic cough.

Description: For lung weakness, it improves breathing, eliminates shortness of breath. An excellent formula for those who smoke or who have smoked either tobacco or marijuana because it helps to repair the damage caused by heat and smoke. For anyone who has a chronic cough or who is easily winded. It strengthens the function of the lungs and can be used long term by anyone who has lung deficiency.

I have not visited this factory and cannot address issues of quality control. It probably contains artificial food coloring. This product has not been tested for drugs or artificial colors. I know of no counterfeits of this product. I have not visited this factory.

Dosage: 4 to 6 pills three times per day.

LONG DAN XIE GAN WAN

Lung Tan Xie Gan Pills
Gentiana Purge Liver Pills
Kwangchow Pharmaceutical Industry Co.
Guangzhou, Guangdong

Note: This product is very popular and there may be counterfeits. I have seen at least three different versions of it.

Common Usage: Liver problems, liver heat, liver fire.

Description: It is very effective in dealing with liver fire which is very common in the U.S. and is usually caused by stress. Its most prominent symptoms include irritability, mood swings, and anger. For a more complete description see page 87.

I recommend the formula produced by Lanzhou Foci Pharmaceutical Company in Lanzhou, China, because it has been tested and has been found to contain no drugs or synthetic chemicals.

Dosage: 8 pills three times per day.

MA HSING CHIH KE PIEN

Ephedra and Apricot Pit Stop Cough Pills
[Based on: Ma Xing Shi Gan Tang]
Discussion of Cold-Induced Disorders
(Shang Han Lun)
Dr. Chang Chung-Ching, 142–220 A.D.
Siping Pharmaceutical Works

Common Usage: Common cold with wheezing.

Description: This is a treatment for a common cold which has developed into a cough and asthma. It clears lung infections and helps to eliminate yellow phlegm trapped in the lungs which causes wheezing.

There may be counterfeits of this product on the market. It has been tested and contains a synthetic drug—ephedrine. It may also contain synthetic dyes. I have not visited this factory.

Dosage: 4 pills three times per day.

MARGARITE ACNE PILLS

Cai Feng Zhen Zhu An Chuang Wan
Colorful Phoenix Precious Pearl Hide Pimple Pills
Modern Formula
Guangdong Foshan Manufactory Corporation, Foshan

Common Usage: Acne.

Description: This product contains pearl powder which is used because a pearl itself is very smooth and smoothes the skin. The herbs in this formula are very cold and clear internal heat. Most acne is caused by internal heat which is generated, especially in young people, by overactive hormones and eating damp, greasy food. Diet is especially important in controlling acne, and it is advisable to avoid fried foods, oily foods and "fast" foods which are of low nutritional quality.

I have not visited this factory and therefore cannot vouch for its quality of production. Samples of this product have been tested and have been shown to contain a pharmaceutical drug.

There is a Plum Flower version which contains no drugs or artificial colors.

Dosage: 6 pills two times per day.

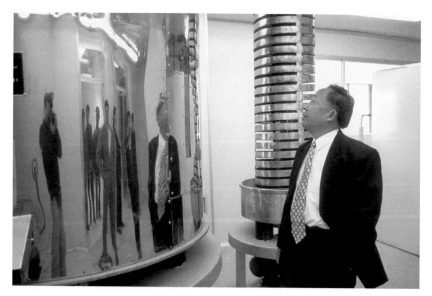

New equipment, Lanzhou

MING MU SHANG CHING PIAN

Brighten Eyes Upper Clearing Heat Pills
Modern Formula
[Based on: Huang Lian Jie Du Wan]
Coptis Clear Toxins Pills
Arcane Essentials from the Imperial Library
(Wai Tai Bi Yao)
Dr. Wang Tao, 752 A.D.
Tianjin Drug Manufactory, Tianjin, China

Common Usage: Conjunctivitis, red eyes.

Description: This product treats acute eye conditions such as conjunctivitis (red, itching, and swollen eyes) and chronic problems such as red eyes from the uprising of liver fire. Under stress, heat accumulates in the liver and rises to affect the eyes and head. This formula clears heat from the liver and reduces itching, tearing, and redness in the eyes.

Note: This product is produced by a high-quality factory with excellent production facilities. I can highly recommend it—but caution you to avoid purchasing counterfeit or smuggled versions of this product.

It has not been tested. I don't believe that it contains drugs or artificial colors.

Dosage: 4 pills two times per day.

PE MIN KAN WAN

Bi Min Gan Wan
Nose Allergy Pills
[Based on: Cang Er Zi San]
Xanthium Powder
Formulas to Aid the Living
(Ji Sheng Fan)
Dr. Yan Yong-He, 1253 A.D.
Chung Lien Drug Works, Wuchang, Hubei Province

Warning: Beware of counterfeits. This product is probably the most widely copied of all Chinese medicines. See page 38 for photo of different packages.

Common Usage: Allergies, nasal congestion.

Description: This is a very popular product in China and in the U.S. It dries phlegm and opens nasal passages, eliminating stuffy nose, sneezing and allergies. It can be taken long term during allergy season to eliminate or reduce the symptoms of hay fever and other allergic reactions. It can also be taken to supplement cold formulas to clear the nose of stuffiness and mucus.

There are so many versions of this formula that it is impossible to know which one is the original. No one that I have spoken with knows which is manufactured by a legitimate factory. It is almost safe to assume that everything on the market is counterfeit and of questionable quality. Some versions have been tested and contain synthetic green dye as well as three pharmaceutical drugs: chlorpheniramine, acetaminophen and phenylpropanolamine hydrochloride.

Plum Flower Brand produces the only version I'm aware of that does not contain drugs, dyes or other chemicals.

Dosage: Most products recommend 3 to 5 pills three times per day.

PING CHUAN PILLS

Stop Asthma Pills
[Based on: Ding Chuan Tang]
Stop Asthma Formula
Exquisite Formulas for Fostering Longevity
(Fu Shou Jing Fan)
Dr. Wu Min, 1530 A.D.
Sing-Kyn Drug House, Guangzhou, Guangdong Province

Common Usage: Relieves the symptoms of wheezing and asthma.

Description: Helps to clear phlegm and heat that contribute to wheezing. See Ding Chuan Wan, page 148.

Test results indicate that this product contains no drugs. I have not visited this factory, so I cannot vouch for the quality of this product. I have not seen any counterfeit versions of it.

Dosage: 10 pills three times per day.

PROSTATE GLAND PILLS

Qian Lie Xian Wan
Modern Formula
Wai Yeung District Medicine Company, Guangdong Province

Common Usage: Reduces prostate enlargement.

Description: This product reduces inflammation, shrinks swollen tissue, regulates urinary function and normalizes male sexual function, a very common problem among men over the age of 40. When the prostate enlarges, it blocks the urethra and slows or stops the flow of urine from the bladder. This formula reduces inflammation in the prostate so that urine flow can normalize or at least improve.

I have not been to this factory and cannot vouch for the quality of production or purity of ingredients. It has not been tested.

Dosage: 5 pills three times per day.

QI YE LIAN ANALGESIC PILLS

Tian Qi (San Qi) Leaf Stop Pain Pills
Notoginseng Leaf Pills
Heping Pharmaceutical Factory, Guangdong Province

Common Usage: Stops Pain.

Description: This is a single herb product intended to stop pain. It is analgesic and has anodyne properties of relieving pain. It can be used for many different aches and pains—arthritis, headache, sciatica, trigeminal neuralgia, carpal tunnel syndrome, and other types of physical discomfort, both external and internal.

It doesn't, however, work like aspirin to alleviate pain immediately. Generally, it takes a few days to feel positive effects.

It has not been tested, and I have not visited this factory.

Dosage: 4 pills three times per day.

REISHI MUSHROOM SUPREME

Reishi-Astragalus Compound
Planetary Formulas

Common Usage: Boosts the immune system.

Description: Please see Astra 8 and Astragalus 10 above, page 223. Both *Ling Zhi (Reishi;* ganoderma) and *Huang Qi* (astragalus) have been proven in clinical tests to elevate the immune system.

I have visited the factory. It contains no drugs or synthetic color.

Dosage: 2 tablets two or three times per day.

SAI MEI AN

Made by Sai Mei An Factory
Modern Formula
Sai Mei An Pharmaceutical Manufactory
Guangzhou, China

Common Usage: Ulcers.

Description: A very effective treatment for ulcers. The herbs in this formula coat the stomach to stop pain and encourage healing. It also neutralizes excess stomach acid which irritates the stomach lining and causes ulcers. It aids the regeneration of the tissue of the stomach lining. It can also be applied topically on open sores to encourage healing. I have seen this product used very effectively in the clinic with positive results.

I have not visited the factory and it has not been tested; the gelatin capsule probably contains synthetic red dye.

Dosage: 3 pills three times per day.

SANG CHU YIN PIEN

Sang Ju Yin Wan
Mulberry Leaf and Chrysanthemum Flower Drink Pills
Tianjin Drug Manufactory, Tianjin

Common Usage: Common cold.

Description: Can be used to treat a common cold with sore throat and fever; especially valuable for children. For a more complete description, please see page 175.

The Tianjin version of this product is of high quality. That factory produces some of the best herbal products in China. As far as I know, this formula does not contain drugs, but it has not been tested.

Dosage: 4 to 8 pills three times per day.

SCIATICA PILLS

Shuo Gu Shen Jin Tong Wan

Common Usage: Sciatica, lower back pain, arthritis.

Description: This formula contains herbs that strengthen the lower back and nourish the kidneys, which controls the lower back. It helps restore normal kidney function and improves low back pain, discomfort, and arthritic conditions. It fortifies the lumbar area where sciatica is initiated.

It has not been tested and I have not visited this factory.

Dosage: 10 pills three times per day.

SHEN LING BAI ZHU PIAN

Ginseng, Poria and Atractylodes Pills
Imperial Grace Formulary of the Tai Ping Era
(Tai Ping Hui Min He Ji Ju Fang)
Imperial Medical Department, 1078–1085 A.D.
Xian Drug Pharmaceutical Works, Xian, Shanxii Province

Common Usage: Improves digestion.

Description: This is a classic herb formula designed to improve digestion especially when dampness is present. This formula can be taken long term to improve digestive function and to drain dampness that slows digestion and interferes with proper digestive function. It treats spleen Qi deficiency affected by dampness which can cause loose stool or diarrhea. I often recommend this formula in the clinic because digestive complaints are very common in a society where we drink lots of ice cold drinks and eat ice cream and salads.

For a more complete discussion of the theory behind this product, please see *Si Jun Zi Tang Wan* (Four Gentlemen Formula), page 178.

I have not visited this factory, but this product has been tested and contains no drugs. It does contain synthetic food coloring.

Plum Flower Brand produces a version of this formula; it is manufactured by the same factory, but it does not contain synthetic food coloring. It is sugar coated.

Dosage: 6 to 12 pills two times per day.

SHENG FA CAPSULES

Hair Growth Capsules
Tianjin Drug Manufactory, Tianjin

Common Usage: Restores hair loss.

Description: In Chinese Medicine, hair is said to be an outgrowth of blood and is controlled by the kidneys. Hair loss is associated with depression, tension or stress, overexertion, or physical debility which exhausts the blood. This formula nourishes blood, improves digestion and assimilation, and strengthens the kidney function.

It has not been tested and I have not visited this factory.

Dosage: 4 capsules two times per day for a period of three to four months.

SHI HU YE GUANG WAN

Dendrobii Night Sight Pills
Formulas from Experience from the Rui Zhu Tang Pharmacy
(Rui Zhu Tang Jing Yan Fang)
Yuan Dynasty, 1279–1368 A.D.

Common Usage: Loss of vision, dry eyes, photophobia.

Description: A formula to strengthen eyesight and to help normalize vision. For those losing their night vision or for those developing tunnel vision. It builds both the liver and the kidneys which support the eyes.

This product has not been tested for drugs. I have seen several versions of this formula, and they may all be legitimate products. I can't tell if there are counterfeits.

Dosage: 5 pills three times per day

SHOU WU CHIH

Polygonum Multiflori Liquid
Modern Formula
United Drug Manufactory, Guangzhou

Common Usage: Darkens hair, improves energy.

Description: This product is primarily a liver tonic for men. It restores normal hair color for those who are turning grey. It strengthens tendons, benefits the eyes, and nourishes blood, replenishing Qi and vital essence which is lost in excessive sexual indulgence. It can be taken long term.

I have seen several counterfeits of this product. It has not been tested, nor have I visited the factory.

Plum Flower has a high-quality version of this product called Shou Wu Tonic Essence which is manufactured in a GMP-certified factory. I have visited the Pangaoshou factory which produces the Plum Flower version and was favorably impressed with the facility. Please see photos of this factory on pages 134, 155, 165, 195.

Dosage: 2 to 3 tablespoons three times per day.

SHOU WU PIAN

Polygonum Multiflori Pills
Black Hair Pills
Modern Formula
Shanghai Medical Works, Shanghai

Common Usage: Darkens hair color, lifts energy.

Description: A single-herb formula, He Shou Wu is reputed to be the herb of choice for restoration of normal hair color. It supposedly reverses the greying process that occurs with aging. There are many formulas available including a Chinese shampoo which promises to restore natural hair color. Because this herb builds the blood, it also improves energy levels.

Shou Wu Pian has not been tested and may contain synthetic dyes.

Plum Flower Brand has a version of this formula which contains no drugs or synthetic dyes.

Dosage: 5 pills three times per day.

SPECIFIC LUMBAGLIN

Te Xiao Yao Tong Lin
Special Efficacy Lower Back Pain Pills
Modern Formula
Guangzhou Pharmaceutical Industrial Corporation

Common Usage: Low back pain.

Description: A terrific formula for lower back pain, weak legs and knees. It can be used for any type of low back pain, sciatica, lumbago, etc.

It has been tested and does not contain any pharmaceutical drugs. I haven't visited this factory, so I cannot verify its quality. The formula does seem to be very effective, and I often recommend it in my practice.

Dosage: 1 to 2 pills three times per day.

STOMACH COOLING

Modern Formula
Shen Herbal Products

Common Usage: Mouth sores, bad breath.

Description: Reduces excessive appetite and bad breath. Other symptoms include mouth sores, burning epigastrium, constipation, painful, swollen gums, a bitter taste in the mouth, and excessive thirst.

I have visited the manufacturing facility. This product has not been tested, but I doubt that it contains drugs or synthetic dyes.

Dosage: 3 to 6 pills two times per day.

STRONG BI YAN WAN

Specific Rhinitis Capsules
Kwang Chow Pharmaceutical Industry Corporation

Common Usage: Allergies, hay fever, nasal congestion.

Description: Like Bi Yan Pian and Pe Min Kan Wan, Strong Bi Yan Wan is used in the treatment of nasal congestion, allergies and hay fever. It can be used to supplement any common cold formula such as Yin Qiao Jie Du Pian or Gan Mao Ling to reduce phlegm blockage in the sinus cavities.

It has not been tested and I have not visited the factory.

Dosage: 1 to 2 capsules three times per day.

SUAN ZAO REN TANG WAN

Jujube Date Tea Pills
Essentials from the Golden Cabinet
(Jin Gui Yao Lue)
Dr. Chang Chung-Ching, 142–220 A.D.
Sing-Kyn Drug House, Guangzhou

Common Usage: Insomnia.

Description: This prescription nourishes the liver, calms the heart, and clears heat from the liver to sedate the mind, encouraging the eyes to close. In Chinese Medicine, it is said that wood (liver) nourishes fire (heart). If the liver is imbalanced, it can affect the heart and therefore the mind, causing mental disturbance, anxiety and insomnia. This formula cools liver heat and nourishes liver blood to cool the liver and relieve stress, allowing peaceful sleep.

I have not visited this factory, but this product has been tested and contains no drugs. It probably does not contain synthetic dyes.

Dosage: To relieve stress 2 to 3 three times per day; For insomnia 2 to 3 one half hour before bedtime as needed.

SUPERIOR SORE THROAT POWDER

Shang Liao Hou Feng San
High-Quality Throat Wind Powder
Fitshan Hang Chun Medicine Factory
Guangzhou, Guangdong

Common Usage: Sore throat.

Description: A powder spray which when applied topically reduces the pain and irritation of sore throat. It can also be used for mouth sores and tongue ulcers.

It has not been tested. I have not visited this factory and cannot vouch for its quality.

Dosage: 1 to 2 sprays in mouth as needed.

TIAN MA MI HUAN SU

Gastrodia Fungus Concentrate Pills
Modern Formula
Fujian Provincial Medicines and Health Products

Common Usage: Lowers blood pressure, migraine headaches.

Description: It lowers blood pressure, sedates the mind and spirit, reduces ear ringing and insomnia caused by excess liver Qi that rises up to the head to cause disturbance. It can also be taken to reduce the symptoms of numbness, muscle spasms, and seizures. It is also very effective in reducing the effects of a migraine headache, but in order to be effective it must be taken long term.

I have not visited this factory.

I have seen two versions of this product. I don't believe that there are any counterfeits of it, but it has not been tested. The sugar-coated tablets appear to contain synthetic dye.

Dosage: 3 to 5 pills three times per day.

TO JING WAN

Tong Jing Wan
Regulate Menses Pills
Modern Formula
China National Chemical Import and Export Co.
Hangzhou, Zhejiang

Special Warning: Do not take during pregnancy; this product could cause miscarriage.

Common Usage: Starts menses.

Description: Breaks up blood stagnation. It is often used to start the menses in women who commonly have clots, irregular periods, difficulty starting periods, or excessively long periods. It can also help eliminate cramps that occur before the start of a period.

It has not been tested. I have not visited the factory and cannot verify its quality.

Plum Flower Brand offers a similar product: Tong Jing Wan, see page 184.

Dosage: 20 pills two times per day.

TRISNAKE ANTI-ITCHING PILLS

Three Snakes Anti-Itching Pills
San She Jie Yang Wan
United Medicine Manufactory, Guangzhou

Common Usage: Itching skin.

Description: This product can be used for any condition which includes itching skin such as skin rash, poison oak, dermatitis, eczema, etc.

I have not visited this factory. I cannot vouch for the quality and purity of this product. It has not been tested.

Dosage: 5 pills three times per day.

WEI TE LING

Stomach Special Remedy
Modern Formula
Tsingtao Medicine Works, Tsingtao

Common Usage: Heartburn, upset stomach.

Description: It reduces hyperacidity of the stomach, stops stomach ache, helps to heal stomach and duodenal ulcers, and stops burping, hiccup and heartburn. It also helps to eliminate gas, bloating and pain. I have found this product to be extremely effective and I have gotten very positive results with my patients.

I have not visited this factory.

I have not seen any counterfeits of this product. It has not been tested to determine if it contains drugs or synthetic dyes.

Dosage: 4 to 6 pills three times per day or as needed.

WU CHIH PAI FENG WAN

Black Chicken Pills
Book for the Protection of Vital Energy for Long Life
(Shou Shi Bau Yuan)
Author Unknown, Ming Dynasty, 1368–1644 A.D.

Common Usage: Builds blood, regulates menses.

Description: Like Ba Zhen Wan (see page 55), this formula for women helps to produce Qi and blood which are lost in menstruation. It supposedly contains a special type chicken for the building of blood as well as many of the herbs found in Ba Zhen Wan. It regulates the menstrual cycle and works to produce normal flow. This is one of the most popular products for women in China. It can be taken every day of the month, but it should be used with caution during menses because it may cause excessive bleeding.

There are many versions of this formula produced by many different factories, none of which has been tested.

I recommend the Plum Flower Brand product because it is guaranteed to contain no drugs or synthetic dyes.

Dosage: 5 small pills three times per day; one large pill per day.

YU NAN BAI YAO

Yunan Province White Medicine
Traditional Family Formula
Yunan Paiyao Factory, Yunan

Special Warning: Do not take during pregnancy.

Common Usage: Stops bleeding, heals injuries, stops pain.

Description: This is the best product available to stop bleeding from cuts or other external trauma. It can be applied directly to a cut or wound to stop bleeding, and it can be taken orally to heal internal bleeding or hemorrhaging from internal injuries. It is an excellent emergency medicine. See page 183 for a more complete description of the effects of *San Qi* (panax notoginseng root).

It is said that Yu Nan Pai Yao is a special family formula which has been kept secret by family members for hundreds of years. It states on the label that it contains 100% San Qi, but the formula probably contains additional herbs.

I have not seen counterfeits of this product. To my knowledge, it has not been tested for drugs or synthetic dyes.

Dosage: 1 to 2 caps four times per day.

ZHONG GAN LING

Valuable Cold Remedy
Modern Formula
Meizhou City Pharmaceutical Manufactory
Guangdong, China

Note: This product has been recently banned in California because it contains synthetic drugs.

Common Usage: Severe common cold symptoms.

Description: For severe common cold which comes on suddenly with fever, sore throat, swollen lymph glands, headache and cough. Use if Gan Mao Ling or Yin Qiao Jie Du Pian have been ineffective.

Zong Gan Ling has been tested and contains three pharmaceutical drugs and synthetic red dye.

There is a version available from Dr. Shen's Formulas.

Dosage: 4 to 6 pills three or four times per day.

9

ABOUT HUMAN RIGHTS

In the last several years, the National press has written a lot of material about human rights abuses in China. It is said in newspaper and magazine articles that some factories in China use slave labor and that working conditions in China are oppressive and sub-standard. It has been reported that workers are exploited, mistreated, and underpaid.

It is also said that the Chinese government is intolerant of dissent and opposes freedom of speech.

Furthermore, some people object to the occupation of Tibet by Chinese forces. I am well aware of these issues, having in the past visited Tibetan refugee centers in Ladakh and Darjeeling, but these are larger political issues outside the scope of this book. I feel that it is only appropriate for me to comment on my own personal observations in China.

Having visited a large number of factories in China over the last ten years, I can honestly say that I have never seen the abusive working conditions described by the news media. In each and every factory, I have had the opportunity to personally interact with workers and to carefully observe their working conditions. Wages are below those in the U.S., but my friends who live in China tell me that they are doing okay because housing and food are relatively inexpensive there. In my opinion, Chinese workers seem to have an increasing amount of disposable income to spend on consumer goods.

I believe it is clear from the pictures in this book that the factories which I have visited are clean and the conditions under which people work are safe and sane.

While I haven't inspected any of the housing units provided by the factories, I have seen them from the outside. I have also visited a number of Chinese friends and their families in their homes. Private housing seems to be in poorer condition than factory housing, which is adequate, safe, and clean.

In short, the working conditions in the factories that I have visited seem to compare quite favorably with conditions in the U.S. I must report that I have seen the very best factories in China, factories as mentioned earlier that have been Internationally certified GMP. Consequently, they are the best China has to offer.

There may be factories that I haven't seen which are substandard, perhaps even abusive. I would have to visit every factory and every facility in China in order to provide a comprehensive view of working conditions in that country. I can only talk about what I have seen.

If you buy the products listed in Chapters 5, 6, and 7 or any Plum Flower Brand product, you can be assured that you are buying the highest quality products from factories which do not violate fundamental human rights. For those who are concerned with these issues, buying high-quality products from factories that treat their employees well is an important message to send to those companies that exploit their employees. You will know at the very least that the money you spend is not supporting oppressive working conditions.

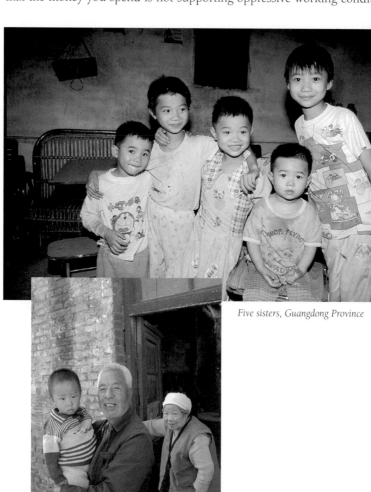

Five sisters, Guangdong Province

Chinese family, Anguo

FOOTNOTES

CHAPTER 1

1. Kluger, Jeffrey, "Mr. Natural," *Time,* 12 May 1997, p. 74.
2. Griggs, Barbara, *Green Pharmacy,* Healing Arts Press, 1981, p. 262.
3. Taylor, Michael, "The Dietary Supplement Debate of 1993: an FDA Perspective," Annual Meeting Federation of American Societies for Experimental Biology, 31 March 1993, pp. 4–5.
4. Ni Maoshing, *The Yellow Emperor's Classic of Medicine,* Shambhala Press, 1995, p. 38.
5. *Time,* p. 74.
6. Wolfe, Sidney, et al, *Pills That Don't Work,* Farrar Straus Giroux, 1981, pp. 1–2.
7. Ibid., pp. 2–3.
8. Hewitt, Paul, *Conceptual Physics,* HarperCollins [sic], 1993, p. 8.
9. Ibid., p. 8.
10. Payer, Lynn, *Medicine and Culture,* Penguin Books, 1988, p. 32.
11. Ibid., p. 149.
12. Ibid., p. 24.
13. Unschuld, Paul, *Medicine in China,* University of California Press, 1986, pp. 274–275.
14. Ibid., pp. 274–275.
15. Payer, p. 26.
16. Ibid., p. 25.
17. Ibid., p. 26.
18. Ibid., p. 130.
19. Ibid., p. 130.
20. Ibid., 51.
21. Ibid., p. 33.
22. Larry King Live, CNN, 1992.
23. Acupuncture Committee, Laws and Regulations Relating to the Practice of Acupuncture, Office of California Department of Consumer Affairs, 1996, p. 2.
24. Mitchell, Barbara, *Acupuncture and Oriental Medicine Laws,* National Acupuncture Foundation, 1997, p. 57.
25. Xie Zhu-Fan, *Best of Traditional Chinese Medicine,* New World Press, 1995, p. 1.
26. Hewitt, p. 8.
27. *Time,* p. 74.
28. Fulder, Stephen and Blackwood, John, *Garlic: Nature's Original Remedy,* Healing Arts Press, 1991, p. 49.
29. Bensky, Dan and Gamble, Andrew, *Materia Medica,* Eastland Press, 1993, p. 441.

30. Bensky, p. 531.
31. Bensky, pp. 441–443.
32. Foster, Steven, *Echinacea: Nature's Immune Enhancer,* Healing Arts Press, 1991, p. 39.
33. Ibid., p. 39.
34. Ibid., p. 68.
35. Ibid., p. 25.
36. Payer, Lynn, *Disease-Mongers,* John Wiley & Sons, Inc., 1992, p. 55.
37. Ibid., p. 55.
38. *Time,* p. 74.
39. Hewitt, p. 8.
40. Beck, James, An open letter to Senator Paul Simon, 1991, p. 6.
41. Ibid., p. 6.
42. Ibid., p. 6.
43. Powers, Francis, An open letter to Congressman George Gekas, 1991, p. 2.
44. See below for references and studies.
45. Bensky, Dan and Barolet, Randall, *Chinese Herbal Medicine: Formulas and Strategies,* Eastland Press, 1990, p. 236.
46. Dr. Xie Zhu-Fan, pp. 93–106.
47. Unschuld, p. 286.
48. Ibid., p. 286.
49. Dr. Zhu Jia-Xing, *Shanghai TCM Journal,* Vol. II, 1995, p. 11.
50. Dr. Xie Zhu-Fan, pp. 93–106.
51. Ibid., pp. 93–106.
52. Ibid., pp. 93–106.
53. Starr, Paul, *The Social Transformation of American Medicine,* Basic Books, 1982, p.123.
54. Payer, Lynn, *Disease-Mongers,* John Wiley and Sons, 1992, p. 19.
55. Ibid., p. 39.
56. Foster, p. 31.
57. Unschuld, p. 274.
58. Powers, p. 1.

CHAPTER 2

59. Dharmananda, Subhuti, Ph.d., *Drugs in Imported Chinese Herb Products,* Institute for Traditional Medicine, Portland, Oregon, November 1996.

GLOSSARY

BLOOD DEFICIENCY

Blood deficiency refers to a lower than optimal level of blood, including red blood cells, white blood cells, fluid volume of blood, and the nutrients carried by the blood. In Western diagnosis, doctors tend to focus only on specific aspects of blood, such as red blood cell count as a measurement of anemia or excessive white blood cell count as an indication of leukemia. The symptoms of blood deficiency occur when the body doesn't produce enough blood or doesn't replace blood lost to external factors, such as excess menstrual bleeding or an injury causing blood loss. Some of the symptoms of blood deficiency are muscle spasms, twitching, dry eyes, dry nails, dry hair, blurry vision and dizziness that occurs when not enough blood is produced to nourish brain cells.

BLOOD STAGNATION

A restriction in normal movement of the blood. A bruise, for example, is localized stagnant blood. Stagnation of blood can occur when the arteries are occluded by atherosclerosis, constricting the normal flow of blood. Blood can also stagnate because of stress. Tension in the body restricts the normal, healthy free flow of blood and Qi. A heart attack or cerebral vascular accident (stroke) are extreme examples blood stagnation. Both occur because the natural flow of blood is literally blocked, causing damage to the cells which are not therefore properly nourished by the blood. The movement of blood can also be impeded by heat and dampness that cause a swelling in localized areas—a type of inflammation—which restricts the movement of Qi and body fluids, including blood.

CHANNELS (OR MERIDIANS)

These are pathways of energy in the body. They have been known for centuries in the Orient, and charts of the meridians can be purchased from suppliers that carry Chinese medical texts.

COLD

This usually refers to the external climate and how it affects the body. But, some people do not generate as much internal heat as others; they may suffer from internal cold or Yang deficiency. Cold can obviously affect an individual who is exposed to extremely chilly weather (hypothermia; frostbite). Overexposure to cold can be very detrimental. Although not as obvious, the fire of life (the vital life force energy) wanes as we age and people can cool down on the inside. Internal cold or Yang deficiency can be an indication of the need for treatment.

DAMP HEAT

When dampness accumulates, it can remain stuck for a considerable time in some people. Long-term conditions of dampness block the free flow of Qi in the body, which then accumulates and forms heat. Damp heat can affect various parts of the body, especially the area around the waist (the lower burner). An accumulation of damp-heat in the lower burner, for example, can cause enlargement of the prostate gland in men or damp-heat can overflow as in vaginal discharge in women.

DAMPNESS

We require fluids (Yin to balance Yang), but excess body fluids (dampness) overwhelm yang energy, dulling the fire of life, making us sluggish. Dampness can be obvious (edema) or it can be seemingly invisible. Normally, our bodies hold an ideal amount of fluid, but each individual cell can absorb excess fluids that sometimes cannot be measured or even seen. Any amount of fluid in excess of normal would be considered dampness. Substantial dampness can be seen as bloating, puffy, swollen ankles or inflamed joints that restrict the range of motion. Insubstantial dampness can show up as digestive difficulties or subjective menstrual problems such as bloating, cramps, and leukorrhea. Exposure to rainy, wet weather can also negatively affect an individual, causing arthritic conditions such as stiffness and pain.

DEFICIENCY HEAT (YIN DEFICIENCY HEAT)

In a healthy body, a balance exists between Yin (essential body fluids) and Yang (life force fire). When the Yin fluids are insufficient, they cannot properly control heat. If we burn out our vital body fluids by being overactive or eating hot, spicy foods, for example, heat appears, especially in the upper body, neck, face and head. Yin deficiency heat can manifest as high blood pressure (Yang excess rising up) or as hot flashes (heat rising up to the face) during menopause.

FIRE

Excessive heat (fire) is generated internally by several different means. The stagnation of Qi in one area of the body, especially in the liver, creates heat. When we are under a great deal of stress, the liver constricts and traps heat that can grow to become fire. This fire can then rise up, for example, to affect the head with such symptoms as headache, burning red eyes, and ear ringing.

HEAT AND TOXINS

When someone gets an infection from a bite or a cut, for example, the infection can penetrate deeper into the body. We see redness, heat, loss of function, pain, and swelling. In TCM, we say that heat has entered the blood, causing the pulse to become rapid. To treat this condition, we cool the blood and clear toxins generated by the infection.

JING (VITAL ESSENCE)

The actual material substance which constitutes the vital life force or the essence of vitality found in sperm and eggs. The Chinese think of this substance as the life force. An individual with a strong constitution has plenty of Jing, while those who are sickly and weak, especially as children, have a deficiency of Jing.

KIDNEYS

The repository of life force energy, the kidneys form the congenital foundation of life, considered our bank account of vitality. In Chinese Medicine, the kidneys are of fundamental importance, because those with strong kidney energy have a strong life force energy; those with weak kidneys are often not healthy. As we age, our kidney energy declines and we lose vitality.

LIVER

In Chinese Medicine, the liver controls the free flow of Qi in the body and is easily affected by emotions which constrict the flow of Qi. In Western Medicine, the liver filters blood and produces bile, its literal mechanical duties, but Chinese medical theory is concerned primarily with the functions of the liver, which are controlling tendons, influencing the eyes, and affecting menstruation.

PHLEGM

Accumulated dampness congeals to become phlegm—thick, sticky dampness that is difficult to remove from the body. We all know how difficult it is to clear phlegm from our nose or our lungs, but phlegm also can manifest in other parts of the body as well. It can be found as fatty deposits in the blood vessels and in the brain (arteriosclerosis). It can be found in lumps and masses such as tumors. Phlegm itself is odorless and relatively colorless, but phlegm plus heat is yellow, thick and smelly.

QI

Although it cannot be seen, touched or smelled, Qi is like electricity. Qi is the energy that drives life. Every food has its essential Qi, like caloric content, that is burned by the body to provide energy. Each individual organ has its own Qi, such as Heart Qi or Lung Qi. When the Qi is weak, the normal function of an organ declines and we say that there is Spleen Qi deficiency or Kidney Qi deficiency, depending on the organ affected. In the body, there are many types of Qi: the Qi of the meridians, the Qi of different areas of the body—Zhong Qi (Central Qi), Qing Qi (Chest Qi).

SHEN (SPIRIT OR HEART)

This concept refers to the life force spirit of each person. Some people have a great deal of vitality while others seem to have little enthusiasm for life. Shen is often thought of as the mental readiness to react to the events of life. People who are dull lack Shen or the spirit of life. Those who are alive and vital have good Shen. Shen is closely associated with the functions of the heart.

SPLEEN

This refers to the entire digestive process and includes the digestive functions of the liver, gallbladder, stomach, pancreas, spleen, and duodenum. Spleen does not refer literally to the organ itself, but to the entire process of digestion. As part of the concept of spleen, the stomach is compared to a cauldron which is used to cook the food. When we eat too much cold food or ice cold drinks, we cool the fire in the cauldron, and the result can be loose, watery stools with undigested food particles (literally undigested food).

TRIPLE BURNER (TRIPLE WARMER)

This concept incorporates all the internal organs into one system. The upper burner refers to the area above the diaphragm and includes the lungs, heart, chest and head. The middle burner refers to the spleen and stomach, the area between the diaphragm and the navel. The lower burner refers generally to the area below the navel, the small and large intestine, kidney, bladder, and sex organs and usually includes liver and gallbladder (though some people put them in the middle burner). The lower burner also includes the legs, knees, ankles and feet. The function of the triple burner is to move fluids (by means of the water passages) throughout the torso and to integrate the functions of all internal organs.

WEI QI

The force field of the body that protects us from foreign invaders. When the Wei Qi is strong, individuals don't catch colds, but when Wei Qi is weak we are vulnerable to colds, allergies, and sickness—wind-borne diseases. Wei Qi provides our resistance to disease and protects us from the wind.

WIND

This is a difficult concept for western minds because wind cannot be seen; it is immaterial. We can see the actions of wind when trees move and we can feel it blowing, but we cannot see it. This is the nature of wind: indefinite, changeable, and wandering. In our bodies, wind can move internally, causing abnormal movement of body parts, such as twitching, muscle spasms, and other abnormal movement like deviation of the eyes. In extreme cases, such as with meningitis, the neck will contort backwards. We say this is caused by extreme heat creating internal wind. Internal wind can manifest in many different ways, but a cerebral vascular accident is called a wind-stroke in Chinese Medicine and often manifests in abnormal movement in the body (paralysis). Most often, pain that moves around in the body from place to place is associated with wind.

WIND-HEAT/WIND-COLD
This is the common terminology for the two main types of common cold. Wind carries the external invading pathogens (bacteria; virus) and can manifest differently in different people. Some people will get chills, body aches, clear or white mucus, and a stiff neck (wind-cold), while some will get predominant fever, sore throat, yellow mucus, and red eyes (wind-heat). There are several other types of colds, but they are not as common and are more difficult to diagnose.

YANG
One of the two basic energies in the universe. Yang energy is the fire of life. It is the energy that animates people—their warmth, vitality and excitement. People who are manic and little children who are hyper are Yang excess, while those who are weak, dull, and sluggish have deficient Yang energy. Yin and Yang ideally work together in harmony to maintain a balance between the forces of fire and water. Too much fire will evaporate water; too much water will put out the fire. We must have both in order to be alive. In our culture, there seems to be a prejudice in favor of Yang energy (youthfulness; loud music; hyperactivity) and it seems to be valued more than Yin (quiet groundedness; thoughtful contemplation), but Yin cannot exist without Yang; nor can Yang exist without Yin.

YIN
Yin is the opposite of Yang—the two basic life force energies. Yin is substance; it is the ground while Yang is the sky. Yin is the green grass flowing across a prairie field; it is the snow capped mountains; it is the vast blue ocean. People with excess Yang are overly excitable, cannot sit still, and seem to go incessantly. But they flame themselves out through excessive action, a fire that consumes the wood too quickly. Without Yin to ground and nurture us, we would float off into the cosmos.

SELECTED BIBLIOGRAPHY

Best of Traditional Chinese Medicine, Zhu-Fan Xie, New World Press, Beijing, China, 1995.

Chinese Herbal Medicine, Formulas and Strategies, Dan Bensky and Randall Barolet, Eastland Press, Seattle, Washington, 1990.

Chinese Herbal Medicine, Materia Medica, Revised Edition, Dan Bensky and Andrew Gamble, Eastland Press, Seattle, Washington, 1993.

Chinese Herbal Patent Formulas, A Practical Guide, Jake Fratkin, Shya Publications, Boulder, Colorado, 1986.

Clinical Handbook of Chinese Prepared Medicines, Chun-Han Zhu, Paradigm Publications, Brookline, Massachusetts, 1989.

Discussion of Cold Induced Disorders (Shang Han Lun), Chang Chung-Ching, 142–220 A.D., edited by Hong-yen Hsu and William Peacher, Keats Publishing, New Canaan, Connecticut, 1981.

The English-Chinese Encyclopedia of Practical Traditional Chinese Medicine, Volume 3, Pharmacology of Traditional Medical Formulae, Chief Editor Xiang-cai Xu, Higher Education Press, Beijing, China, 1990.

The English-Chinese Encyclopedia of Practical Traditional Chinese Medicine, Volume 5, Commonly Used Chinese Patent Medicines, Chief Editor Xiang-cai Xu, Higher Education Press, Beijing, China, 1990.

Handbook of Chinese Herbal Formulas, Him-che Yeung, Institute of Chinese Medicine, Second Edition, Rosemead, California, 1995.

Outline Guide to Chinese Herbal Patent Medicines in Pill Form, An Introduction to Chinese Herbal Medicines, Margaret Naeser, Boston Chinese Medicine, Boston, Massachusetts, 1990.

The Web That Has No Weaver, Understanding Chinese Medicine, Ted Kaptchuk, St. Martin's Press, 1986.

The Yellow Emperor's Classic of Medicine (Neijing Suwen), Anonymous, 220 A.D., translated by Maoshing Ni, Shambhala Press, Boston, Massachusetts, 1995.

APPENDIX 1

AMERICAN MANUFACTURERS OF CHINESE HERBAL PRODUCTS

There are a number of American companies which are now marketing Chinese herbal products. These companies produce quality products which are based on many of the classical Chinese formulas that I have already discussed in this book.

DR. SHEN'S FORMULAS
Shen Herbal Products
908 Ensenada
Berkeley, CA 94707
510-527-HERB

HEALTH CONCERNS
8001 Capwell Dr.
Oakland, CA 94621
510-639-0280

K'AN HERB COMPANY
6001 Butler Lane
Scotts Valley, CA 95066
800-543-5233

PLANETARY HERBS
19 Janis Way
Scotts Valley, CA 95066
800-606-6226

SEVEN FORESTS
Institute for Traditional Medicine
2017 SE Hawthorn
Portland, OR 97214
800-544-7504

APPENDIX 2

CHINESE HERB SUPPLIERS

MAYWAY
1338 Mandela Parkway
Oakland, CA 94607
800-262-9929

NU HERBS
3820 Penniman Ave.
Oakland, CA 94619
800-233-4307

SPRING WIND
(Licensed Practitioners Only)
2325 4th St., Suite #6
Berkeley, CA 94710
510-849-1820

SUPERIOR TRADING COMPANY
837 Washington St.
San Francisco, CA 94108
415-982-8722

TAI SANG
1018 Stockton St.
San Francisco, CA 94108
415-981-5364

APPENDIX 3

DOCUMENTS OF GMP CERTIFICATION

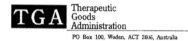

TGA Therapeutic Goods Administration
PO Box 100, Woden, ACT 2606, Australia

COMMONWEALTH
DEPARTMENT OF
HEALTH AND
FAMILY SERVICES

Certificate of Good Manufacturing Practice

Lanzhou Foci Pharmaceutical Company Ltd, 336 Yanchang Road, Lanzhou City, Gansu, P.R. China has been subject to a Good Manufacturing Practice (GMP) audit by an officer of the GMP Audit & Licensing Section, Conformity Assessment Branch, Therapeutic Goods Administration.

From the knowledge gained during this audit on 23rd and 26th August 1996, it is considered that the company has an overall acceptable level of compliance with the Australian Code of Good Manufacturing Practice for Medicinal Products which encompasses all the recommendations of the World Health Organisation in relation to GMP.

This certificate is issued in respect of the manufacture of non-sterile herbal medicines intended for supply in Australia.

This certificate is not issued under the WHO Certification Scheme but is a statement of the manufacturing standard of the company.

This certificate remains valid until September 1999.

Signed

Date 4/9/96

R W Tribe
Chief GMP Auditor

Certificate No 448

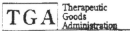 **TGA** Therapeutic
Goods
Administration
PO Box 100, Woden, ACT 2606, Australia

Commonwealth Department of
Health and
Family Services

Certificate of Good
Manufacturing Compliance

This is to certify that Guangzhou Pangaoshou Pharmaceutical Co Ltd, of Dong Shen Industry District, Shiqiao, Panyu, Guandong, P R CHINA, has been subject to a Good Manufacturing Practice (GMP) audit by officers of the GMP Audit & Licensing Section, Conformity Assessment Branch, Therapeutic Goods Administration, (TGA). The TGA is part of the Australian Department of Health and Family Services. Australia is a signatory to the Pharmaceutical Inspection Convention (PIC).

From the knowledge gained during this audit of Guangzhou Pangaoshou Pharmaceutical Co Ltd, the latest of which was conducted on 4th July 1996, it is considered that the company complies with the requirements of the current Australian Code of Good Manufacturing Practice for Therapeutic Goods Medicinal Products which encompasses all the recommendations of the World Health Organisation in relation to GMP.

The company is authorised to manufacture non-sterile chinese herbal medicines in the form of lozenges and liquid herbal preparations for oral use, derived from aqueous/alcoholic extracts of herbs.

This certificate is not issued under the WHO Certification Scheme but is a statement of the quality standard of the factory.
This certificate remains valid until November 1998.

Signed

Date 19/12/96.

R W Tribe
Chief GMP Auditor
GMP Audit & Licensing Section   Certificate No. 488
Conformity Assessment Branch

TGA	Therapeutic Goods Administration

PO Box 100, Woden, ACT 2606, Australia

Certificate of Good Manufacturing Practice

Commonwealth Department
Health and
Family Services

Guangzhou Qixing Pharmaceutical Co. Ltd, 33 ChiGang Bei Road, XinGang Road Central, Guangzhou P.R. China has been subject to a Good Manufacturing Practice (GMP) audit by an officer of the GMP Audit & Licensing Section, Conformity Assessment Branch, Therapeutic Goods Administration.

From the knowledge gained during this audit conducted on 26 and 27th November, 1996 it is considered that the company has an overall acceptable level of compliance with the Australian Code of Good Manufacturing Practice for Medicianal Products which encompasses all the recommendations of the World Health Organisation in relation to GMP.

This certificate is issued in respect of the manufacture of non-sterile herbal medicines (in tablet, pill, capsule, granule and powder form) intended for supply in Australia.

This certificate is not issued under the WHO Certification Scheme but is a statement of the quality standard of the company.

This certificate remains valid until November 1999.

Signed

Date . 9/12/96

R W Tribe
Chief GMP Auditor
GMP Audit & Licensing Section   Certificate No: 472
Conformity Assessment Branch

PRACTICAL APPLICATION OF FORMULAS TO SPECIFIC SYMPTOMS AND DISORDERS

ABDOMINAL DISCOMFORT (STOMACH UPSET)
Mild pain, fullness, bloating, gas, traveler's diarrhea.

Bao He Wan: similar actions as Po Chai Pills and Pill Curing, with fewer herbs; can be taken long term. p. 60.

Bao Ji Wan: for temporary relief of stomach discomfort; very similar to Curing Pills. p. 223.

Pill Curing (Kan Ning Wan): for temporary relief of stomach fullness after a big meal; especially useful after family meals like Thanksgiving and Christmas. Can also be taken for mild cases of food poisoning or for stomach flu. Also any temporary stomach discomfort. p. 230.

Po Chai Pills: the same as Bao Ji Wan. p. 223.

Shu Gan Wan: for treating a condition called liver attacking spleen; for the effects of stress on digestion, in particular bloating and upper abdominal discomfort with symptoms of belching, acid regurgitation, or the feeling of food stuck in the upper abdomen. p. 102.

Xiao Jian Zhong Wan: for stomach upset caused by poor digestion, especially when cold foods or cold drinks aggravate the condition. p. 193.

ABSCESS, SKIN: BOILS, CARBUNCLES
Skin problems, sores, skin eruptions.

Ba Zhen Wan: for chronic sores that will not heal; provides the proper nutrition to speed up the healing process. p. 55.

Lian Qiao Bai Du Pian (Lien Chiao Pai Tu Pien): for skin rash, poison oak, and skin conditions characterized by heat, redness, swelling and discomfort. Also for boils, carbuncles, etc. p. 217.

Shi Quan Da Bu Wan: similar to Ba Zhen Wan; for deficiency of Qi and blood which prevents sores from healing; also for those with cold hands and feet who are extremely deficient. p. 101.

Wu Wei Xiao Du Yin: heals sores on the skin, acute boils, carbuncles, sores with swelling, heat, pain, and redness. p. 190.

ACNE

Usually occurring in adolescents with poor diets, but also associated with hormone imbalance; it is best to avoid greasy, oily food; hot, spicy food; fried foods, barbecue, smoked meats etc. Green tea is a welcome addition to the diet.

Margarite Acne Pills: for mild adolescent acne. p. 240.

Wu Wei Xiao Du Yin: clears up blemishes, infectious acne, and extreme swelling as well as red sores. p. 190.

AGING

The study of the aging process in Chinese Medicine finds its roots in the ancient practices of Taoist priests who lived in the mountains and practiced breathing meditation and dietary restrictions designed to extend life. Their practices have continued since before the Tang Dynasty (8th Century). An important part of their ritual and practice was the study of herbs to increase longevity and to slow the aging process. The fascination with herbal prescriptions to increase longevity continues in China today. Below, you will find some basic prescriptions based on Taoist medicine which are aimed at slowing the aging process and increasing vitality.

Ba Ji Yin Yang Wan: slows the aging process, restores youthful energy by strengthening various organ functions, especially the kidneys which in Chinese medicine are the repository of genetic Qi. p. 133.

Gu Ben Wan: replenishes essential vital life force energy necessary to slow the aging process and improve everyday life. p. 75.

Hai Ma Bu Shen Wan: a broad spectrum tonic aimed at restoring basic organ functions and replenishing Qi, essentially restoring the life force fire. p. 159.

Huan Shao Wan (Return to Youth): a prescription targeting restoration of youthful energy and vitality. p. 161.

AIDS

There are a number of modern formulas manufactured primarily in the U.S. which seek to boost weakened immune systems. They are all similar in content, consisting primarily of the chief herbs Huang Qi (astragalus root) and Ling Zhi (reishi; ganoderma mushroom). The supporting herbs vary with different formulas, but all attempt to elevate the immune system. Modern research in China has shown that the herbs used in these formulas boost immunity by increasing levels of T Cells and B Cells.

Astra 8: builds the immune system and resistance to disease. p. 223.

Astragalus 10: similar to Astra 8 above. p. 223.

Reishi Mushroom Supreme: similar to the formulas above. p. 244.

ALLERGIES

Hay fever, sneezing, red eyes, and irritation of the nose are all symptoms of allergic reaction to pollens and dust. The best way to treat allergies is to prevent them in the first place by building up the immune system, using Jade Screen (Yu Ping Feng San Wan; see below). In Chinese Medicine, allergies and common colds occur when the immune system is weak. It is said that the Wei Qi (protective Qi) is deficient and doesn't protect the body from wind-borne invasion.

Bi Yan Pian: dries nasal passages, eliminates phlegm and mucus.p. 224.

Pe Min Kan Wan: similar to Bi Yan Pian; dries phlegm, clears the nasal passages. p. 242.

Xin Yi Wan: similar to Bi Yan Pian and Pe Min Kan Wan; opens the nasal passages and dries excess phlegm and dampness from the sinuses. p. 196.

Yu Ping Feng San: the best formula for preventing allergies. It can be taken alone or with other prescriptions to strengthen the immune system. Over-the-counter homeopathic remedies are also very effective for short-term relief of allergies. p. 201.

ALOPECIA

Hair loss, probably caused by genetic predisposition or stress which interferes with digestion and reduces the body's ability to produce blood and Qi which nourish hair.

Gui Pi Wan: builds blood and Qi to properly nourish hair. p. 76.

Sheng Fa: for restoring normal hair growth. p. 247.

Shou Wu Pian: a single-herb formula for restoring normal hair color and for restoration of hair loss. He Shou Wu is an herb which builds blood and nourishes the hair. p. 248.

AMENORRHEA

Absence of menstruation; anyone attempting to remedy this condition must be certain that the woman being considered is not pregnant.

Special Warning: not having a menstrual period can be an indication of pregnancy.

Si Wu Tang Wan (Four Substances Formula): a four-herb formula for building and invigorating blood. Can help begin the menstrual cycle for those who are either weak, pale and tired or who have mild clots and purple blood at the beginning of their period. p. 179.

Tao Hong Si Wu Tang Wan: this formula contains the same herbs as Si Wu Tang Wan, but with additional herbs to break up blood stagnation. It can be used by women who have heavy, purple clots during their menstrual cycle or no period at all because of blood stagnation. Symptoms include severe pain and cramping before menses, along with more emotional disharmony. p. 180.

To Jing Wan: a very strong formula to start menses; do not take if pregnant. p. 252.

Tong Jing Wan: this formula can be used to start menses for women who are late and should be expecting their cycle to start, but it should not be used by those who are anemic or weak. It should not be used by anyone who is pregnant. p. 184.

ANEMIA

Iron deficiency is the most common cause of anemia in the world. It is especially prevalent in countries with a predominantly rice diet, which doesn't include enough meat. Vegetarians in the U.S., especially women, can become anemic because they are not replacing iron lost in menstrual blood. There are some very good iron supplements sold in health food stores, such as Floradix Iron and Herbs. I recommend staying away from iron supplements sold in drug stores. These often contain ferrous sulfate which is very difficult for the body to assimilate and can cause constipation, because the iron is not readily absorbed in the digestive tract and ends up being passed out of the body in the feces. Ferrous Sulfate is low quality and an extremely cheap form of iron. Iron supplements can cause very serious stomach pain, so they should be taken with meals or after eating. Floradix Iron and Herbs does not usually cause stomach upset. To enhance its effectiveness, I also recommend one of a number of green foods, such as spirulina, chlorella, or blue-green algae. Green foods contain chlorophyll which is almost identical to a hemoglobin molecule. Taken with iron, chlorophyll has all the constituents to build blood.

Ba Zhen Wan: builds both blood and Qi, and is a classic formula to nourish and promote good health in women. p. 55.

Gui Pi Wan: contains many blood building herbs; elevates both Qi and blood, especially for those who are engaged in excessive mental activities such as studying or for those involved in intense mental work as in the computer industry. p. 76.

Si Jun Zi Tang Wan (Four Gentlemen): improves digestion; when digestion improves, the body's ability to build red blood cells improves. p. 178.

Si Wu Tang Wan: half of the above formula, Ba Zhen Wan; contains herbs to build healthy blood and to keep blood from becoming stagnant. p. 179.

Tang Kwei Gin: builds healthy blood; classic formula for women in a pleasant tasting liquid. Similar to Ba Zhen Wan. p. 212.

Wu Chih Pai Feng Wan (Black Chicken Pills): similar to Ba Zhen Wan with a black feathered chicken added to improve the blood-building effects of the herbs. p. 253.

Xiang Sha Liu Jun Zi Tang Wan (Six Gentlemen): improves digestion; similar to Si Jun Zi Tang Wan, plus additional herbs. p. 111.

ANGINA

Heart or chest pain; this is a very serious condition. Anyone with chest pains should see a doctor immediately. Other symptoms include tight chest, stuffy breathing, pain radiating down the left arm.

Dan Shen Pian: opens coronary arteries to allow blood to flow more freely to the heart muscle. p. 231.

Dan Shen Yin Wan: this formula relieves tightness in the chest and encourages blood flow to the heart. p. 147.

Sheng Mai San: improves circulation, stops palpitations, mental restlessness, dry mouth, dry throat, thirst, and night sweats. p. 177.

Xue Fu Zhu Yu Tang (Stasis in the Mansion of Blood): breaks up stagnant blood in the chest, reduces chest pain. p. 197.

ANOREXIA

Loss of appetite; inability to eat and thrive. Sometimes psychosomatic, but often occurs because of weak digestion.

Bao He Wan: eliminates stuffy, full feeling after eating, improves digestion and assimilation. p. 60.

Ren Shen Jian Pi Wan: for those with very weak digestion who are emaciated, cannot put on weight, listless, easily fatigued with a small appetite. p. 97.

Xiang Sha Yang Wei Wan: improves digestion, encourages weight gain among the excessively thin. p. 112.

ANXIETY

An Shen Bu Xin Dan: natural tranquilizer to reduce depression and anxiety which is associated with internal heat that rises up to disturb the heart and mind. p. 54.

Bai Zi Yang Xin Wan: calms and relaxes the heart and mind. p. 59.

Ban Xia Hou Po Wan: for stress and the feeling of something stuck in the throat. This is not an uncommon sensation and is treated as a psychosomatic disease by Western doctors. p. 136.

Chai Hu Long Gu Mu Li Wan: for anger, irritability, and an irregular heartbeat along with a feeling of fullness or tightness in the chest. p. 143.

Gan Mai Da Zao Wan: can be taken by menopausal women who suffer from mood swings, uncontrollable emotions and stressful, unstable behavior. p. 154.

Gui Pi Wan: nourishes blood and calms the heart. It is especially good for the student syndrome of over-studying and spending too much time thinking and worrying. p. 76.

Jia Wei Xiao Yao Wan: reduces stress and anxiety in patients with signs of internal heat, PMS symptoms, anger and irritability. p. 166.

Tian Wang Bu Xin Dan: helps anxiety associated with mental restlessness. Other symptoms can include dry mouth, dry throat, palpitations, hot flashes or heat rising up to the face, and nightsweats. p. 108.

Xiao Yao Wan: reduces stress, PMS symptoms, and the blues. p. 116.

APOPLEXY (POST-STROKE)
Paralysis of one side of the body after a cerebral vascular accident or stroke.

Bu Yang Huan Wu Tang Wan: improves function of paralyzed limbs, opens channels so that Qi can flow to heal paralysis, atrophy and cellular damage. p. 141.

Tian Ma Gou Teng Wan: eliminates spasms, tremors, and other abnormal movements of the body. p. 181.

APPENDICITIS
See a doctor immediately.

APPETITE, POOR

Bao He Wan: treats food stagnation or poor appetite caused by food being stuck in the stomach and not descending properly. p. 60.

Ren Shen Jian Pi Wan: also warms digestive fire; improves assimilation and harmony in the stomach and digestive organs. p. 97.

Si Jun Zi Tang Wan: the principle formula in all of Chinese medicine for improving digestion. Please see the accompanying article in the back of the book which discusses this formula. p. 178.

Xiang Sha Liu Jun Zi Wan: a variation of Si Jun Zi Wan with more herbs to regulate digestive energy as well as nourish and improve digestion. p. 111.

Xiang Sha Yang Wei Wan: focuses more on improving stomach function while the above formula focuses on the spleen. p. 112.

Xiao Jian Zhong Wan: another variation of Four Gentlemen; it warms digestive fire more strongly than Si Jun Zi Tang Wan. p. 193.

ARTHRITIS

Du Huo Ji Sheng Wan: especially good for the elderly or for those who suffer from aches and pains, especially low back and knee pain. p. 150.

Guan Ji Yan Wan: also known as Joint Inflammation Pills. p. 157.

Fang Ji Huang Qi Wan: for arthritic conditions in which there is inflammation and edema of the skin. p. 153.

Tian Ma Wan: a formula for minor aches and pains. p. 106.

Xiao Huo Luo Dan: a very hot formula, but very useful; for individuals who suffer from cold, painful arthritis which is worse in the morning. p. 192.

ASTHMA
Wheezing, difficulty inhaling oxygen.

Ding Chuan Wan: a terrific formula for reducing wheezing. I have seen most asthma patients improve dramatically after about a month of using this product. p. 148.

Er Chen Wan: clears excess phlegm that is either white or clear and should be used only when excess phlegm is the cause of wheezing. p. 71.

Ma Hsing Chih Ke Pien: for yellow phlegm stagnation in the lungs with associated wheezing; for secondary stages of a common cold. p. 238.

Ping Chuan Pills: similar to Ding Chuan Pills. p. 148.

Qing Qi Hua Tan Wan: for excess phlegm which is sticky, yellow and is causing wheezing. p. 96.

BACK PAIN, LOW BACK PAIN

Duo Huo Ji Sheng Wan: strengthens the body by nourishing blood and digestion to feed the muscles and eliminate pain; for low back pain, sore knees and ankles. p. 150.

Specific Lumbaglin: one of the best products for treating low back pain; can be taken long term. p. 249.

BAD BREATH

Stomach Cooling: cools excessive heat in the stomach which can rise up and affect the breath. p. 249.

BEDWETTING

Jin Suo Gu Jing Wan: for weakness of the kidneys and incontinence. p. 84.

BELCHING

Shu Gan Wan: for belching associated with stress; helps reduce stagnation of Qi in the liver which causes belching. p. 102.

BLADDER INFECTION

Ba Zheng San: clears heat and inflammation which can cause burning, scanty yellow urination and pain. Encourages normal function of the urinary system. p. 135.

Bi Xie Fen Qing Wan: difficult, cloudy, troubled urination. p. 137.

Chuan Xin Lian: natural antibiotic, treats all types of infections, including bladder infections. Very effective combined with Ba Zheng San. p. 228.

BLOATING, STOMACH FULLNESS

Bao He Wan: eliminates food stagnation in the stomach; the feeling of being stuffed after eating. p. 60.

Curing Pills, Bao Ji Wan, Po Chai Pills: all reduce stomach discomfort of all types. pp. 223, 230.

Shu Gan Wan: for bloating associated with stress. p. 102.

BLOOD POISONING (SEPTICEMIA)

Huang Lian Jie Du Wan: a natural antibiotic for any type of infection. p. 163.

BLOOD PRESSURE, HIGH

Compound Cortex Eucommia Tablets: contains herbs which have been proven in clinical studies in China to reduce blood pressure. p. 229.

Hawthorn Fat-Reducing Pills: reduces cholesterol dramatically by reducing fat in the blood stream to reduce blood pressure. p. 234.

Tian Ma Gou Teng Wan: can be used long term to reduce the causes of high blood pressure which are not recognized by western-style doctors. p. 181.

BOILS

Huang Lian Jie Du Wan: for all types of skin infections, boils, carbuncles, that are red and inflamed with pus. p. 163.

Huang Lian Shang Ching Pian: for any type of skin eruption with red, inflamed skin with pus. p. 216.

Wu Wei Xiao Du Yin: for any type skin infection with heat, redness, swelling and discomfort. p. 190.

BREATH, SHORTNESS OF BREATH

Ding Chuan Wan: treats shortness of breath and wheezing. p. 148.

Jie Geng Wan: a single-herb formula for chronic cough and chronic shortness of breath. Strengthens the function of the lungs. p. 81.

Li Fei Tang Yi Pian: strengthens the lungs; improves lung function. p. 238.

BRONCHITIS

Ching Fei Yi Huo Pien: a terrific formula for yellow, sticky, thick, yellow phlegm in the lungs. pp. 216, 227.

Er Chen Wan: use for clear or white, thick, copious phlegm trapped in the lungs. p. 71.

Qing Qi Hua Tan Wan: for yellow sticky phlegm or copious thick yellow phlegm which has invaded the lungs or the bronchials. p. 96.

CANCER

Treatment of this condition is the subject of a book all by itself. I cannot recommend any particular formula to treat cancer. Please see a licensed practitioner.

CARBUNCLES, BOILS

Wu Wei Xiao Du Yin Wan: for any skin infection with heat, redness, swelling and discomfort. p. 190.

CHEST PAINS, TIGHT CHEST

Chen Xiang Hua Qi Wan: for the feeling of a tight, constricted chest which makes breathing difficult and affects the heart. p. 64.

Dan Shen Pills: see angina above. p. 231.

Dan Shen Yin Wan: for mild angina pain which is not life threatening. For persistent pain accompanied by shortness of breath or other breathing difficulties, see a licensed practitioner. p. 147.

Xue Fu Zhu Yu Tang Wan (Stasis in the Mansion of Blood): breaks up blood stagnation in the chest; in Chinese medicine, pain is always caused by stagnation. p. 197.

CHOLESTEROL

Hawthorn Fat-Reducing Pills: dramatically reduces fat deposits in the blood. p. 234.

Tian Ma Gou Teng Yin: see high blood pressure above. p. 181.

COMMON COLD

There are several different types of common colds in Chinese Medicine. In order to treat a condition effectively, you must have a correct diagnosis. The two most prevalent types of common colds are wind-cold and wind-heat. Gan Mao Ling is the only formula that treats both types of common cold.

Chuan Xiong Cha Tiao Wan: wind-cold type common cold with headache. p. 65.

Da Chai Hu Wan: treats a common cold that is getting worse and starting to invade the deeper levels of the body. p. 145.

Fang Feng Tong Sheng San: common cold that lingers on the surface of the body, neither improving nor getting too much worse. p. 151.

Gan Mao Ling: treats common cold. p. 219.

Ge Gen Wan: for wind-cold type common cold with stiff neck. p. 156.

Huo Xiang Zheng Qi Wan: stomach flu. p. 78.

Sang Chu Yin Pien: same as Sang Ju Yin Wan. pp. 174, 244.

Sang Ju Yin Wan: for wind-heat type common cold; a milder version of Yin Qiao, useful for children. pp. 174, 244.

Yin Qiao Jie Du Pian: a very common treatment for wind-heat type common cold with sore throat, fever and other heat symptoms. pp. 121, 214.

Yu Ping Feng San Wan: an immune system booster to prevent common colds and allergies. p. 201.

CONCUSSION

Xue Fu Zhu Yu Tang: breaks up blood stagnation, bruising, and other damage from brain trauma. Before using this formula, make certain that all internal bleeding has stopped. p. 197.

CONJUNCTIVITIS

Ming Mu Shang Ching Pian: for more serious conjunctivitis. p. 240.

Sang Ju Yin Wan: for mild conjunctivitis accompanying a common cold; especially for children. pp. 174, 244.

CONSTIPATION

Da Huang Jiang Zhi Wan: a strong purgative; for severe cases of constipation. p. 146.

Fructus Persica Tea Pills (Peach Kernel Tea Pills): aka: Tao Ren Wan; Run Chang Wan; a mild laxative. p. 105.

Ma Zi Ren Wan: a mild laxative. p. 89.

Peach Kernel Tea Pills: aka Tao Ren Wan, Run Chang Wan, Fructus Persica: another mild laxative. p. 105.

Tong Shun Wan: a mild laxative. p. 186.

Wu Ren Wan: a mild laxative. p. 105.

CONTUSIONS, BRUISES, SPRAINS, STRAINS

Jin Gu Die Shang Wan (The Great Mender): for sprains, strains, bruises, contusions, injuries of all types. p. 168.

The Great Mender: see Jin Gu Die Shang Wan above. p. 168.

Yu Nan Bai Yao: for injuries, bleeding, and trauma. p. 254.

COUGH

Bai He Gu Jin Wan: for chronic cough with weakness of lungs and kidneys. Strengthens both organ systems to eliminate coughing. p. 57.

Er Chen Wan: stops cough caused by white or clear phlegm. p. 71.

Fritillaria and Loquat Cough Syrup: a thinner cough syrup; good for children. p. 211.

Jie Geng Wan: chronic cough. p. 81.

Loquat Flavored Jelly: a thick cough syrup that will relieve symptoms of mild cough. p. 211.

Mai Wei Di Huang Wan: for chronic cough, especially smoker's cough associated with heat in the lungs. p. 90.

Ning Sou Wan: stops chronic and acute cough. p. 172.

Qing Qi Hua Tan Wan (Clean Air Tea Pills): stops cough associated with yellow phlegm. p. 96.

San She Dan Chuan Bei Ye: for coughs and yellow phlegm, bronchitis, emphysema, or asthma; good for children. p. 211.

DEPRESSION

An Shen Bu Xin Dan: anxiety and depression. p. 54.

Jia Wei Xiao Yao Wan: reduces stress with PMS symptoms, anger, and irritability p. 166.

Shu Gan Wan: reduces stress and depression. p. 102.

Xiao Yao Wan: reduces stress, depression and PMS symptoms. p. 116.

DIABETES

Diabetes is very difficult to treat; some people simply cannot be helped except by insulin injections. Others can improve by changing their diet and adhering to a strict regimen of exercise and food restrictions. It is not recommended to self-treat this condition.

Yu Quan Wan: for mild symptoms and to reduce dependence on insulin; should only be used in conjunction with seeing a licensed practitioner. p. 202.

DIARRHEA

Bu Zhong Yi Qi Wan (chronic): for weak digestion leading to chronic loose stools; western-style doctors do not understand that an individual can have diarrhea without a bacterial infestation. p. 62.

Huang Lian Jie Du Wan (acute with fever): for diarrhea with accompanying fever and/or chills and fever, more severe than simply acute diarrhea. p. 163.

Huang Lian Su Wan (acute): bacterial diarrhea, traveler's diarrhea, Delhi belly, food poisoning, etc. Widely popular in China. pp. 165, 235.

Xiang Lian Wan: regulates the bowels and stops diarrhea from mild cases of food poisoning. p. 191.

DIGESTION, POOR

Mu Xiang Shun Qi Wan: irritable bowel syndrome and lower bowel complaints; regulates bowel function. p. 93.

Ping Wei San: strong formula to remove dampness, excess saliva. p. 174.

Ren Shen Jian Pi Wan: improves digestion. p. 97.

Shen Ling Bai Zhu Pian: for poor digestion with accompanying dampness, loose stools, and food stagnation. Very good for those who have sticky, loose stools. p. 246.

Si Jun Zi Wan (Four Gentlemen): the classic formula to improve weak digestion. p. 178.

Xiang Fu Li Zhong Wan: increases digestive fire. p. 110.

Xiang Sha Liu Jun Wan (Six Gentlemen): for poor digestion. p. 111.

Xiang Sha Yang Wei Wan: improves digestion. p. 112.

Zhen Wu Tang Wan: for people who are very weak and almost unable to digest food, low energy, pale, cold, often with watery stools with undigested food. p. 205.

Zi Sheng Wan: a broad-spectrum digestive aid. p. 126.

DIURETIC

Wu Pi Yin Wan: for superficial water retention. p. 188.

DIZZINESS

Can be caused by several different conditions: 1. Blood deficiency: blood does not properly nourish the brain, making the person dull and listless; 2. Phlegm stagnation which interferes with normal brain function, creating foggy thinking; 3. Excess yang rising up to the head which can manifest as internal wind (see glossary) and become vertigo.

Ba Zhen Wan: nourishes blood and strengthens digestion to improve the body's ability to make blood and promote healthy brain function. p. 55.

Du Zhong Pian: reduces high blood pressure and clears the head. p. 229.

Si Wu Tang: tonifies and regulates blood to properly nourish the brain and prevent dizziness. p. 179.

Tian Ma Gou Teng Yin: sedates excess yang and clears phlegm stagnation in the brain. p. 181.

EAR INFECTION

Chuan Xin Lian: natural antibiotic. p. 228.

Huang Lian Jie Du Wan: a natural antibiotic to clear infection especially in the upper body and head. p. 163.

Huang Lian Shang Ching Pian: fights infections in any area of the head or face. Treats sore throat, ear infections, mouth sores, swollen gums, toothache, conjunctivitis, severe infected acne, etc. p. 216.

EAR RINGING

Er Long Zuo Ci Wan (Tso-Tzu Otic): for tinnitus, ear ringing. p. 72.

Long Dan Xie Gan Wan: from liver heat and liver fire rising, excess yang energy that rises up to disturb the ears. pp. 87, 238.

Tian Ma Gou Teng Yin: for excess yang uprising. When the yin is deficient, yang rises up and disturbs the hearing. This type of ear ringing is high-pitched and incessant. It will remain after you press against the ear. p. 181.

ECZEMA

This condition is very difficult to treat. I don't believe that there is a good herb formula which would be effective. Please see a licensed acupuncturist. I have not heard positive reports about successful treatment from conventional western-style dermatology. Eczema is usually associated with asthma. In Chinese medicine, the lungs control the skin. When the lungs are weak, the individual is more likely to experience skin disorders. A Chinese doctor would most likely tonify the kidneys and the lungs. Such a treatment might take several months to a few years in order to show significant improvement.

EDEMA

Fang Ji Huang Qi Wan: for sudden, superficial edema on the skin. p. 153.

Wu Pi Yin Wan: for superficial edema of the skin. Also for bloating and accumulation of fluids. p. 188.

EMPHYSEMA

See a licensed practitioner.

EYES, DRY

Ming Mu Di Huang Wan: similar to the above formula. p. 91.

Qi Ju Di Huang Wan: dry eyes can be effectively treated with this formula. Sometimes, it may take a month or more to clear up. p. 95.

EYES, RED

Long Dan Xie Gan Wan: acute red eyes can be the result of excess liver heat which comes from too much stress and is associated with irritability and anger. pp. 87, 239.

Ming Mu Shang Ching Pian: red eyes and inflammation, conjunctivitis. p. 240.

FATIGUE

There are many causes of fatigueóblood deficiency, loss of blood and Qi from childbirth, poor diet, illness, stress. You should seek out a practitioner to determine whether the cause of fatigue is serious, especially if the fatigue is unusual and lasts longer than a few days.

Ba Zhen Wan: almost identical to Shi Quan Da Bu Wan except for the absence of warming herbs. Can be used for blood deficiency after childbirth without heat signs. Women especially should take this formula with an iron supplement and Evening Primrose oil to restore normal blood production and eliminate PMS symptoms. p. 55.

Bu Zhong Yi Qi Wan: improves digestion and lifts energy in a healthy way; for fatigue in women associated with extra long, heavy menses. Or for general fatigue associated with excessive mental activity. p. 62.

Shen Qi Da Bu Wan: for general fatigue of short duration; gently elevates energy without being too warming or too excessive in stimulation. p. 99.

Shen Qi Wu Wei Zi Wan: increases energy and soothes the mind. p. 100.

Shi Quan Da Bu Wan: warming and tonifying; it can be used by anyone experiencing fatigue and cold hands and feet and a pale tongue, especially with small, hard-to-find pulses. p. 101.

Shou Wu Chih: builds blood and restores vitality. p. 248.

Shou Wu Tonic Essence: builds blood and restores vitality. p. 210.

Yang Rong Wan: strengthens a woman's vital functions. p. 118.

Yang Ying Wan: for weakness and debility; increases energy, builds blood, elevates vitality. p. 120.

FEVER, HIGH
See a doctor immediately.

Gan Mao Ling: common cold with slight fever and chills. p. 219.

Huang Lian Jie Du Wan: fever with infection. p. 163.

Yin Qiao Jie Du Wan: mild fever and sore throat with common cold. pp. 121, 214.

FLU
See common cold.

Huo Xiang Zheng Qi Wan: stomach flu. p. 78.

FRACTURES

Jin Gu Die Shang Wan (The Great Mender): heals external trauma and injuries, broken bones, sprains, strains, contusions, bruises, etc. p. 168.

The Great Mender: see above. p. 168.

GALLBLADDER DISEASE

Gallbladder problems such as gallstones, pain in the gall bladder area (below the ribs on the middle right side), stomach discomfort, poor digestion, etc., are very common and are very often treated with surgery. Some individuals with gallbladder problems have a bowel movement immediately after eating. Or they have problems with gas and bloating immediately after meals. Gallbladder problems are not uncommon in our country because stress damages the gallbladder and over time will cause it to malfunction. Commonly found in women over the age of forty.

Li Dan Wan: reduces gallbladder inflammation, helps to eliminate gallbladder discomfort. p. 238.

Long Dan Xie Gan Wan: reduces heat and dampness in the liver, gallbladder, improves gallbladder function. pp. 87, 239.

GASTRITIS (SEE POOR DIGESTION)

Bao He Wan, Bao Ji Wan, Curing Pills: for temporary, minor digestive complaints and stomach discomfort. pp. 60, 223, 230.

GLAUCOMA

Ming Mu Di Huang Wan: reduces pressure in the eye, calms down the liver energy which is directed upward to the eyes. p. 91.

GOITER

Hai Zao Wan: restores normal thyroid function, reduces thyroid swelling. p. 161.

Nei Xiao Lei Li Wan: reduces lumps on the neck. p. 171.

GOUT

This is a very difficult disease to treat. Please see a licensed acupuncturist.

HAIR COLOR

Shou Wu Chih, Shou Wu Pian, Shou Wu Tonic Essence: helps restore normal hair color. In order to be effective, it must be taken long term. pp. 248, 210.

HEADACHES

Headaches are very common and very difficult to treat with herbs alone. I have seen a number of patients improve with acupuncture and herbal treatments; both the duration and the intensity of headaches can diminish over time. It is a process that requires patience and commitment from a patient as well as the practitioner in order to be effective.

In Chinese Medical theory, there are many different types of headaches, each having a different cause and different treatment. You must have a proper diagnosis and proper treatment in order to improve. Self medication probably will be of little benefit. No herbal product offers the immediate relief from pain provided by Aspirin or its cousins, Tylenol and Advil.

If you have developed a headache from an injury and it has not improved or may have gotten worse, see a doctor immediately.

Chuan Xiong Cha Tiao Wan: headache with common cold, plus some other types of headache. p. 65.

Gui Pi Wan: for a headache from blood deficiency; this type of headache is dull and occurs late in the afternoon; or a headache due to over-thinking or excessive worry. p. 76.

Yan Hu Suo Pian: for frontal headache and insomnia. p. 199.

HEADACHES, MIGRAINE

Long Dan Xie Gan Wan: headaches from liver fire. pp. 87, 239.

Tian Ma Gou Teng Yin Wan: headaches on the side of the head or above one eye; usually affects one side of the head at a time; rarely affects both sides at the same time. p. 181.

HEART DISEASE
Any condition affecting the heart can be very serious. It is highly recommended that you seek the help of a health care practitioner in order to treat this condition properly.

Angina Pain
See a licensed practitioner.

Dan Shen Pian: opens coronary arteries and encourages proper blood flow through the heart. p. 231.

Dan Shen Yin Wan: chest pain associated with the heart. p. 147.

Cholesterol, High

Hawthorn Fat-Reducing Pills: reduces cholesterol levels. I have seen this product dramatically reduce blood cholesterol. Taking flax seed oil and fish liver oils is also recommended. p. 234.

Palpitations

Bai Zi Yang Xin Wan: calms the heart, reduces heat in the upper body and eliminates dry mouth, dry throat, heat rising up to the face and neck. p. 59.

Chai Hu Long Gu Mu Li Wan: for palpitations from stress and anxiety. p. 143.

Tian Wang Bu Xin Dan: calms the heart beat, reduces heart stress and soothes the mind. p. 108.

HEMIPLEGIA (PARTIAL PARALYSIS)

Bu Yang Huan Wu Wan: reduces the effects of paralysis; for post-stroke and other causes of paralysis. p. 140.

HEMORRHOIDS

Fargelin (for Piles): shrinks swollen tissue and pulls energy upwards. p. 232.

Fargelin, extra strength: shrinks inflamed tissue and stops pain. p. 232.

HEPATITIS
See a doctor immediately.

Long Dan Xie Gan Wan: can reduce the effects of hepatitis, but hepatitis is a very serious condition and this formula should only be taken in conjunction with treatment from a licensed practitioner. pp. 87, 239.

HERNIA
See a licensed practitioner.

Ji Sheng Ju He Wan: for chronic hernia which is not acute. p. 80.

HERPES

Long Dan Xie Gan Wan: for genital herpes, which is often caused by heat and inflammation moving downward in the liver channel that encircles the genital area. pp. 87, 239.

HYPERTENSION
See Blood Pressure, High.

IMMUNE SYSTEM
There are a number of formulas available to boost immunity, but it has to be done

*long-term and maintained consistently in order to be effective. Our busy life-style cre-
ates stresses that have compromised many individual's immune systems.
Environmental pollution, poisoned food crops, and a poor diet contribute to chronic
illness which is rampant in the U.S.*

Astra 8, Astragalus 10, Reishi Mushroom Supreme: modern formulas made
here in the U.S. specifically for AIDS and cancer patients with weak immune
systems. There are many variations of these formulas made by other companies,
but they all contain Reishi (Ling Zhi) mushrooms and Astragalus (Huang Qi) as
the chief herbs for strengthening the immune system. pp. 223, 244.

Liu Wei Di Huang Wan (Six Flavor Tea Pills): tonifies the kidneys and
improves liver function; for increased production of hormones and building
immune function. Tests in China have demonstrated that this formula is
extremely effective in elevating immune response, including the production of
both B Cells and T Cells. p. 85.

Si Jun Zi Tang Wan (Four Gentlemen): the classic formula for improving digestion. When digestion is optimal, then all the vital nutrients in the diet are
assimilated and therefore available to rebuild cells, maintain cellular integrity
and to produce plenty of healthy Qi. Many studies in China have been performed over the last few years which have proven that Si Jun Zi Tang Wan
boosts the immune system. p. 178.

Yu Ping Feng San (Jade Screen): classic formula for building Wei Qi, the protective energy that guards the body from foreign invasion. p. 201.

INCONTINENCE

Jin Suo Gu Jing Wan: for weakness of the kidneys leading to urinary incontinence. p. 84.

INFECTION

Huang Lian Jie Du Wan: by far the best formula for fighting almost any type of
infection. Modern antibiotics are becoming ineffective in treating some types of
bacterial infections; strains of different bacteria are evolving which are developing immunity to the most powerful pharmaceutical antibiotics available. This
is caused by excessive reliance on common antibiotics and the fact that pharmaceutical antibiotics are single chemical compounds. A formula like Huang
Lian Jie Du Wan most likely will always be effective because it is doubtful that
bacteria can adapt to compounds which are chemically complex. Huang Lian
Jie Du Wan has many active ingredients, making it far too complex for bacteria
to neutralize it. p. 163.

INFERTILITY

Fu Ke Zhong Zi Wan: improves a woman's ability to conceive; warms the womb to create a positive environment for conception. p. 74.

Yang Rong Wan: warms the womb and increases Qi. p. 118.

INFLUENZA
See flu above.

INJURY, TRAUMA

Jin Gu Die Shang Wan (The Great Mender): see below. p. 168.

The Great Mender (Jin Gu Die Shang Wan): fractures, sprains, strains, bruises, etc. p. 168.

Tian Qi Wan: for internal injuries, bruises, cuts, scrapes, contusions. p. 183.

Yu Nan Pai Yao: for any type of external or internal injury. Can be applied topically to cuts and wounds to stop bleeding. p. 254.

INSOMNIA
There are several possible causes of insomnia, among them blood deficiency, Qi deficiency, Yin deficiency, disturbed shen (spirit), excess heat, liver Qi stagnation, internal wind, and several others. Any time insomnia persists longer than a few days, seek the advice of a licensed acupuncturist.

An Mien Pian: quiets the heart and allows the mind to rest. p. 222.

An Shen Bu Xin Wan: calms spirit and encourages a quiet mind. p. 54.

An Shui Wan: calms the mind, encourages sleep. p. 131.

Bai Zi Yang Xing Wan: clears heat from the heart which disturbs the spirit and makes the mind restless. Nourishes the liver to support the heart and the mind. p. 59.

Good Sleeping and Worry Free Tea Pills: soothes the mind and encourages peaceful sleep. p. 234.

Suan Zao Ren Tang Wan: nourishes blood to properly cool the heart and calm the mind. p. 250.

Tian Wang Bu Xin Dan: calms the heart and the mind. p. 108.

IRRITABLE BOWEL SYNDROME

Mu Xiang Shun Qi Wan: regulates bowel function, normalizes the movement of feces in the small intestine and large intestine. p. 93.

JAUNDICE
See your doctor or licensed acupuncturist.

KIDNEY DEFICIENCY

Jin Gui Shen Qi Wan: for the very weak and feeble or for those with congenital weakness of the kidney function. p. 82.

Liu Wei Di Huang Wan: the classic formula for strengthening kidney yin function. p. 85.

You Gui Wan: a variation of Liu Wei Di Huang Wan with warming properties for tonifying kidney yang as well as kidney yin. p. 200.

Zuo Gui Wan: stronger tonifying kidney Yin function than Liu Wei Di Huang Wan. p. 206.

KIDNEY INFECTION (BLADDER INFECTION)
This can be very serious. See a licensed practitioner.

Ba Zheng San: clears heat and inflammation which can cause burning, scanty yellow urination and pain. Encourages normal function of the urinary system. p. 135.

Bi Xie Fen Qing Wan: difficult, cloudy urination. p. 137.

Chuan Xin Lian: natural antibiotic, treats all types of infections. Very effective with Ba Zheng San. p. 228.

LAXATIVES
See constipation.

LEUKORRHEA (VAGINAL DISCHARGE)

Chien Chin Chih Tai Wan: eliminates the source of dampness, regulates menstrual cycle and stops cramps. pp. 215, 226.

Yu Dai Wan: dries wetness, clears heat and inflammation. p. 123.

MENOPAUSE

Da Bu Yin Wan: nourishes vital yin fluids; a stronger treatment for hot flashes or excess heat in the face or upper body than Zhi Bai Di Huang Wan. p. 68.

Er Xian Tang Wan: for such mixed hot and cold symptoms, simultaneous internal heat plus cold hands and feet, low back pain, irritability, depression, shaking, muscle cramps, and other symptoms associated with menopause. p. 232.

Gan Mai Da Zao Wan: treats dry organ syndrome, a Chinese diagnosis of certain internal organs, such as the liver, spleen, and heart, which are being properly nourished with age. This prescription is intended to be taken long term. p. 154.

Two Immortals: see Er Xian Tang Wan above. p. 232.

Zhi Bai Di Huang Wan (Zhi Bai Ba Wei Wan): great for hot flashes, calms anxiety, reduces irritability and anger; extremely popular and very effective. p. 124.

MENSTRUAL PROBLEMS

Blood Deficiency

Ba Zhen Wan: builds blood and regulates the menstrual cycle for those who have small, short periods, or who have cramps and pain after menses. Also for those who experience depression and fatigue after their cycle. p. 55.

Dang Gui Su Wan: regulates menses and builds blood. p. 69.

Dang Gui Wan: improves digestion, builds blood. p. 70.

Shi Quan Da Bu Wan: similar to Ba Zhen Wan above, but with the addition of warmer herbs for those who are experiencing cold symptoms, such as cold hands and feet. p. 101.

Tang Kwei Gin: builds healthy blood, restores regularity to the menstrual cycle. p. 212.

Depression

Xiao Yao Wan: builds blood and regulates stuck liver Qi which results in depression, irritability and mood swings. p. 116.

Depression and Irritability

Jia Wei Xiao Yao Wan: similar to Xiao Yao Wan above, but with stronger herbs to reduce irritability and anger. p. 166.

Excessive Bleeding without Clots

Bu Zhong Yi Qi Wan: for spotting between periods or periods longer than six days with light bleeding and pale blood. p. 62.

Fatigue

Ba Zhen Wan: builds blood and improves energy. p. 55.

Chai Hu Shu Gan Wan: see Shu Gan Wan below. p. 144.

Dang Gui Wan: builds blood to eliminate fatigue. p. 70.

Irregular Menstruation

Wen Jing Tang: for an irregular cycle, difficult menses, with mixed cold and heat sensation. Symptoms include either early or late menses, increased body temperature, especially in the evening along with heat sensation in the face, hot palms and feet, dry mouth, dry throat along with cold abdomen. p. 187.

Menstrual Cramps

Corydalis Yan Hu Suo Pian: stops menstrual cramps and abdominal pain; also effective against headaches associated with the menses. p. 230.

Yan Hu Suo Wan: stops pain; most effective in treating lower abdominal pain and cramping. p. 199.

Miscarriage

See a licensed practitioner; there can be several causes for this condition, especially if it repeats itself. A Chinese doctor specializing in gynecology can be of great assistance.

Yang Rong Wan: strengthens the womb and supports the body's ability to hold a child. If pregnant, please see a licensed practitioner. p. 118.

Morning Sickness

See a licensed practitioner to make certain that the formulas below are appropriate; do not take chances when pregnant with medicine that you do not understand.

Huo Xiang Shun Qi Wan: settles the stomach. p. 78.

Pill Curing: settles upset stomach. p. 230.

Xiang Sha Yang Wei Wan: settles the stomach; improves digestion. p. 112.

PMS

Dang Gui Su Wan: regulates the menses. p. 69.

Dang Gui Wan: improves overall menstrual function, including reducing PMS symptoms. p. 70.

Jia Wei Xiao Yao Wan: reduces PMS symptoms like depression, irritability and anger. p. 166.

Shu Gan Wan: for clots, purple blood and cramps before period, and swollen or tender breasts. p. 102.

Xiao Yao Wan: reduces PMS symptoms like depression. p. 116.

MOTION SICKNESS

Bao Ji Wan (Po Chai Pills): similar to Pill Curing. p. 223.

Huo Xiang Shun Qi Wan: calms and settles the stomach. p. 78.

Pill Curing: the best product to take with any type of upset stomach; settles and smoothes out almost all difficulty. You can also drink ginger tea or take ginger capsules. p. 230.

MOUTH SORES

Stomach Cooling: heat rises up from the stomach and causes swollen gums, mouth sores, and bad breath. p. 249.

MUMPS

See a licensed practitioner.

NASAL CONGESTION

See allergies above.

NAUSEA

Bao Ji Wan (Po Chai Pills): treats nausea from food stagnation or when an individual feels stuffed. p. 223.

Huo Xiang Zheng Qi Wan: see motion sickness above. Most useful for nausea with stomach flu symptoms. p. 78.

Pill Curing: see motion sickness above. This is the most popular common remedy for any type of stomach upset—gas, bloating, nausea, etc. p. 230.

Xiang Fu Li Zhong Wan: treats nausea from eating cold foods. p. 110.

NIGHTSWEATS

Da Bu Yin Wan: for more severe cases of nightsweats and extreme symptoms of menopause. p. 68.

Zhi Bai Ba Wei Wan: the best for treating mild cases of nightsweats and symptoms of menopause. p. 124.

Zhi Bai Di Huang Wan: same as Zhi Bai Ba Wei Wan above. p. 124.

ORGAN PROLAPSE

Bu Zhong Yi Qi Wan: for mild prolapse of stomach, uterus, anus, or intestines. p. 62.

PARALYSIS

Bu Yang Huan Wu Wan: post-stroke partial paralysis. p. 141.

Xiao Huo Luo Dan: for post-stroke, or arthritis that causes numbness and tingling where there is no sign of heat, redness and swelling. p. 192.

PHLEGM

Bi Yan Pian: for nasal congestion and stuffy nose. p. 224.

Er Chen Wan: for clear or white phlegm in the lungs. p. 71.

Ma Hsing Chih Keh Pien: for yellow phlegm in the lungs associated with wheezing. p. 238.

Pe Min Kan Wan: for nasal congestion, mostly with clear phlegm or runny nose associated with allergies. p. 242.

Qing Qi Hua Tan Wan: for yellow phlegm congestion in the lungs and bronchial passages. p. 96.

San She Dan Chuan Bei Ye: for yellow phlegm, bronchitis, or chronic conditions with stubborn yellow phlegm that is hard to eliminate; good for children. p. 212.

PNEUMONIA
See a doctor.

POISON OAK

Armadillo Counter Poison Pills: for skin rash like poison oak, any type of red, inflamed skin problems. p. 222.

Lian Qiao Bai Du Pian: for skin rash caused from allergies or any other type of red, inflamed skin. p. 217.

PROSTATE, ENLARGED
Benign prostate hypertrophy; a very common problem in our society, affecting a majority of men over the age of forty. It is quite treatable with either Chinese remedies or with western herbal treatment. Saw Palmetto extract (serenoa repens) is the treatment of choice in Western Europe and is better than the drugs that are available. It is widely available from health food stores.

Kai Kit Wan: reduces inflammation and clears heat from the area around the genitals. In Chinese medicine, an enlarged prostate is often associated with lower burner damp heat—the accumulation of dampness and heat causes enlargement of internal organs which puts pressure on the urethra, causing blockage. This usually comes from a diet of excessive heat producing foods, such as alcohol, hot spicy meals, and rich fatty foods. p. 236.

Prostate Gland Pills: similar to Kai Kit Wan above. p. 243.

RHEUMATISM
See arthritis.

RHINITIS
See allergies or nasal congestion.

SCIATICA
Characterized by a sharp pain shooting down the back of one thigh or the other from the lower back. In some cases, the pain shoots all the way down to the foot.

Du Huo Ji Sheng Wan: a remedy specifically designed for low back pain and sciatica. p. 150.

Specific Lumbaglin: a product to reduce low back pain and sciatica. p. 249.

SCROFULA
Nei Xiao Lei Li Wan: for reducing lumps on the neck. p. 171.

SEPTICEMIA (AKA BLOOD POISONING)
Any infection in the body in which pathogens invade the blood stream; a systemic infection. See a doctor immediately.

Huang Lian Jie Du Wan: a natural antibiotic, used any time there is infection in the body. It can be used for almost any type of infection. p. 163.

SINUSITIS
See nasal congestion.

SKIN RASH
Armadillo Counter Poison Pills: reduces heat and swelling on the skin; for poison oak or any other type of acute skin rash. p. 222.

Huang Lian Shang Ching Pian: clears heat and inflammation from any type of red, inflamed sore. p. 216.

Lian Qiao Bai Du Pian: reduces heat and inflammation; clears skin. p. 217.

SKIN, ITCHING
Kai Yeung Pills: stops skin itching; for any type of skin condition with associated itching. p. 237.

Tri-Snake Anti-Itching Pills: stops itching; for any type of itching skin, including reactions to drugs, eczema, urticaria, etc. p. 252.

SORE THROAT

The best home remedy that I have found for acute sore throat is apple cider vinegar; to use, dilute three parts water to one part vinegar. Gargle several times a day.

Superior Sore Throat Powder: a spray powder that can be applied to the back of the throat to relieve sore throat pain. p. 251.

Yin Qiao Jie Du Pian: relieves sore throat pain as well as the symptoms of a common cold or flu. pp. 121, 214.

STIFF NECK

Ge Gen Wan: used primarily as a common cold formula with a stiff neck; it can also be taken for stiff neck alone. It is sometimes recommended by chiropractors for this purpose. p. 156.

STROKE

See a licensed practitioner.

SWALLOWING (DIFFICULT)

Ban Xia Hou Po Wan: for difficulty swallowing and the feeling that something is stuck in the throat. p. 136.

SYNCOPE

See a licensed practitioner.

TESTICLES, SWOLLEN

Ji Sheng Ju He Wan: for swelling of testes, especially from stress and extreme emotional upset. p. 80.

THIRST (DRY MOUTH)

Ba Xian Chang Shou Wan: same as Mai Wei Di Huang Wan. p. 90.

Mai Wei Di Huang Wan: for thirst with dry throat, night sweats, ear ringing, dizziness, and dry cough. p. 90.

THROAT, PLUM PIT
The feeling of something stuck in the throat.

Ban Xia Hou Po Wan: for the feeling of something being stuck in the throat, usually caused by stress; difficulty swallowing. p. 136.

THYROID
Hai Zao Wan: for slow thyroid function (hypothyroid). p. 161.

TINNITUS
See ear ringing.

TONSILLITIS
Huang Lien Shang Ching Pian: for any infection, swelling or acute inflammation of the head, neck, or lungs. Includes treating boils, carbuncles and other skin infections. p. 216.

TUBERCULOSIS
See a licensed practitioner.

ULCERS
Sai Mei An: for stomach or duodenal ulcers, or to apply topically to the skin. p. 245.

ULCERS, BLEEDING
Yu Nan Pai Yao: can be taken internally in capsules; heals all types of bleeding conditions, internal or external. Also for cuts, scrapes, abrasions, wounds, etc. p. 254.

UPPER RESPIRATORY TRACT INFECTION
Ching Fei Yi Huo Pian: for thick yellow mucus in the lungs and bronchials. pp. 216, 227.

Ma Hsing Chih Keh Pian: for cough, wheezing, and thick yellow mucus in the lungs and bronchials. p. 238.

Qing Qi Hua Tan Wan: for thick yellow mucus in the lungs, cough and bronchial infection. p. 96.

URETHRITIS (INFLAMED URETHRA)

Ba Zheng San: for urinary tract infections with heat, burning, and discomfort. p. 135.

Bi Xie Fen Qing Wan: for frequent, difficult urination with cloudy or milky-colored discharge in the urine. p. 137.

Long Dan Xie Gan Wan: for painful, difficult urination that is caused by stress. pp. 87, 239.

URINARY TRACT INFECTION

There are several different types of urinary tract infections recognized by Chinese medicine—called lin syndromes. Among them are blood lin, cake lin (cloudy), stone lin, heat lin, and Qi lin. In western medicine, doctors almost always prescribe antibiotics to treat these conditions (except for kidney stones), but antibiotics unfortunately are over-used and cause complicating side effects. It is very common for women to get yeast infections after taking a round of antibiotics. So, Western treatment addresses one problem and creates another. Taking acidophilus in liquid, powder or pill form during and after antibiotics sometimes counteracts the negative effects of antibiotics.

Heat lin: burning, urgent, concentrated, yellow urination with a strong smell. Prescriptions that treat this problem include:

Ba Zheng San: for burning, discomfort and difficult urination. This formula is especially effective when taken with Chuan Xin Lian. p. 135.

Chuan Xin Lian: for burning, painful, and difficult urination. p. 228.

Huang Lian Jie Du Wan: for hot, painful urinary difficulty. p. 163.

Long Dan Xie Gan Wan: for heat and burning urination. pp. 87, 239.

Cake lin or cloudy urine:

Bi Xie Shang Qing Wan: for cloudy, frequent, difficult and milky urine. p. 139.

Blood lin: blood in the urine. If this persists for longer than 24 hours, please see a licensed practitioner. Bleeding can be a sign of a more serious condition.

Ba Zheng San: for burning, discomfort and difficult urination. This formula is especially effective when taken with Chuan Xin Lian. p. 135.

Yu Nan Pai Yao: can be taken internally in capsules; heals all types of bleeding conditions, internal or external. Also for cuts, scrapes, abrasions, wounds, etc. p. 254.

Qi lin: for stress, or difficult, hesitant urination, lower abdominal bloating, fullness and pain.

Shen Ling Bai Zhu Pian: strengthens digestion which controls fluids in the body and helps regulate urination. p. 246.

URINATION, FREQUENT AND CHRONIC
According to Chinese Medicine, men should ideally urinate 3 to 5 times per day while women should urinate 5 to 7 times per day. Any more than this constitutes frequent urination and is usually associated with weakness of the kidney energy.

Liu Wei Di Huang Wan: strengthens the function of the kidneys and reduces the need to urinate as often. It may take several weeks to improve kidney function and to reduce the frequency of urination. It should gradually improve and normalize. p. 85.

Bu Zhong Yi Qi Wan: lifts energy in the center of the body, for weakness and deficiency of Qi. p. 62.

URTICARIA (SKIN RASH)
Armadillo Counter Poison Pills: for poison oak and red skin rash. p. 222.

Kai Yeung Pills: for skin rash and itching skin. p. 237.

Lian Qiao Bai Du Pian: for red, inflamed rashes, any type of skin condition with bumps, boils, carbuncles, etc. p. 217.

UTERINE BLEEDING (ABNORMAL)
Do not ignore this condition; see a licensed practitioner. Uterine bleeding may be a sign of a more serious condition.

Bu Zhong Yi Qi Wan: for spotting between periods or for chronic prolonged periods with light, pale bleeding. p. 62.

VAGINAL DISCHARGE
Chien Chin Chih Tai Wan: eliminates the source of dampness, regulates menstrual cycle and stops cramps. pp. 215, 226.

Yu Dai Wan: dries wetness, clears heat and inflammation. p. 123.

VERTIGO (DIZZINESS)
Gui Pi Wan: for weakness and blood deficiency in which the body is not producing enough blood to properly nourish the brain. p. 76.

Qi Ju Di Huang Wan: for weakness of the kidneys which do not support the liver, allowing excess liver energy to rise up and disturb the brain, causing dizziness. p. 95.

Tian Ma Gou Teng Yin Wan: for excess energy moving to the head, the feeling that the feet are not grounded. p. 181.

VOMITING

Ban Xia Hou Po Wan: for on and off vomiting associated with stress. p. 136.

Bao He Wan: for vomiting associated with food stuck in the stomach and not moving down the digestive tract. p. 60.

Huo Xiang Zheng Qi Wan: for stomach flu type symptoms with associated vomiting. p. 78.

Xiang Fu Li Zhong Wan: for vomiting associated with discomfort after eating cold foods, icy drinks, and ice cream. p. 110.

Xiang Sha Liu Jun Wan: for weak digestion associated with bulimia and anorexia. p. 111.

WEAKNESS, DEBILITY
See also fatigue.

Ching Chun Bao: a temporary energy boost; to keep you going when you are tired. p. 226.

Cong Rong Bu Shen Wan: awakens the fire of life, increases energy. p. 67.

Ge Jie Da Bu Wan: a general tonifying formula to strengthen kidney function and improve energy levels. p. 233.

Shen Qi Da Bu Wan: elevates Qi, increases energy. p. 99.

WHEEZING
See asthma above.

WOUNDS

Tian Qi Wan: for injuries, cuts, scrapes, contusions, etc. p. 183.

Yu Nan Pai Yao: for any kind of puncture, wound, scrape, cuts, contusions, etc. Internal or external. p. 254.

FORMULA INDEX